This book contains three book manuscripts authored by Sammy Parker:

Book 1: Anxiety: Overcome Stress, Panic Attacks, and Fear

Book 2: Anxiety: Free Yourself from Shyness, Constant Worry, and Trepidation

BOOK 3: How to Analyze People: Using Human Psychology to Successfully Analyze and Understand Anyone from Anyplace and Anywhere

Anxiety and How to Analyze People: 3 Manuscripts

Anxiety: Stress, Panic Attacks and Fear

Anxiety: Shyness, Constant Worry, and Trepidation

How to Analyze People: Social Skills, People Skills, Body Language, Relationships, and Nonverbal Cues

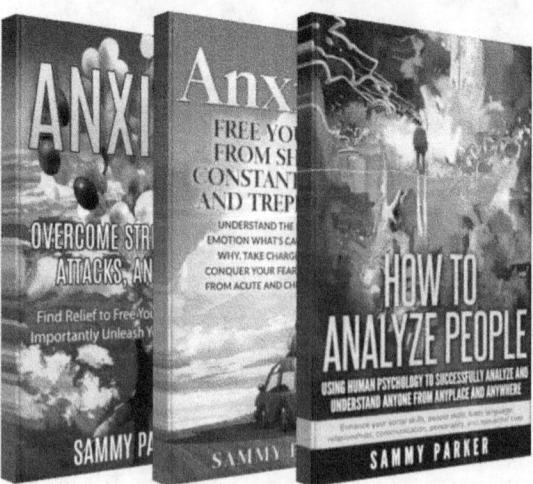

Anxiety:
Overcome Stress, Panic Attacks, and Fear

By Sammy Parker

Find Relief to Free Yourself and Most Importantly <u>Unleash</u> Your Inner Peace

ANXIETY

OVERCOME STRESS, PANIC ATTACKS, AND FEAR.

Find Relief to Free Yourself and Most Importantly Unleash Your Inner Peace

SAMMY PARKER

Introduction

I would like to thank you for downloading the book, *"Anxiety - Overcome Stress, Panic Attacks, and Fear"*.

This book contains proven steps and strategies on how to overcome anxiety, fear and panic attacks.

Anxiety is a widespread problem that has affected the lives of many. If you are a victim of this monstrous condition, your life is probably very chaotic; one thing or the other always flusters you to a point where you never feel settled or relaxed.

This jitteriness adversely affects the quality of your life, your relationships, your professional life, as well as your state of mind; and because anxiety has wrapped its wings around you, you never feel happy, confident, poised, or peaceful.

This is not how your life should be; it is not how you should live your life. You cannot let anxiety control every aspect of your life. You MUST MAKE THE UNEQUIVOCAL CHOICE TO DO SOMETHING.

Fortunately, you can do something about your anxiety. Yes, anxiety is curable however, while big pharmaceutical companies are quick to push this or that pill as the ultimate cure for anxiety, the hidden truth to curing anxiety is one simple word: YOURSELF.

Do not let the anxiety pill adverts brainwash you; you are the only person with the capacity to treat your anxiety permanently.

Are you wondering how to make that possible, how to live an anxiety free life? Well, wonder no more because this book focuses on that specific subject.

This book aims to provide you with proven steps and strategies you can implement to overcome anxiety, unleash your inner peace and self-esteem, and live a successful and fulfilled life. To make this book an easy read, we shall go through a systematic approach guaranteed to help you overcome anxiety.

Thanks again for downloading this book, I hope you enjoy it!

© Copyright 2016 by Sammy Parker - All rights reserved.

This document is geared towards providing exact and reliable information in regards to the topic and issue covered. The publication is sold with the idea that the publisher is not required to render accounting, officially permitted, or otherwise, qualified services. If advice is necessary, legal or professional, a practiced individual in the profession should be ordered.

- From a Declaration of Principles which was accepted and approved equally by a Committee of the American Bar Association and a Committee of Publishers and Associations.

In no way is it legal to reproduce, duplicate, or transmit any part of this document in either electronic means or in printed format. Recording of this publication is strictly prohibited and any storage of this document is not allowed unless with written permission from the publisher. All rights reserved.

The information provided herein is stated to be truthful and consistent, in that any liability, in terms of inattention or otherwise, by any usage or abuse of any policies, processes, or directions contained within is the solitary and utter responsibility of the recipient reader. Under no circumstances will any legal responsibility or blame be held against the publisher for any reparation, damages, or monetary loss due to the information herein, either directly or indirectly.

Respective authors own all copyrights not held by the publisher.

The information herein is offered for informational purposes solely, and is universal as so. The presentation of the information is without contract or any type of guarantee assurance.

The trademarks that are used are without any consent, and the publication of the trademark is without permission or backing by the trademark owner. All trademarks and brands within this book are for clarifying purposes only and are the owned by the owners themselves, not affiliated with this document.

Table of Contents

Step 1: Identify, Accept, and Label Your Anxiety

Step 2: Accept Change Is Progressive and Your Today Does Not Define Your Tomorrow

Step 3: Make Changes and the Right Choices Right Now

   How to Presently Make Positive Changes

   Identify Negative Behaviors That Increase Your Condition And Improve Them

Step 4: Practice Visualization and Anchoring

   Visualize a Peaceful You

   Anchor Peace in Your Mind

Step 5: Be Mindful of Your Blessings, and the Present

   How to Become Conscious of Your Present

Step 6: Practice Regular Meditation

   How to Meditate For Anxiety Relief

Step 7: Be Around Positive People and Spread Happiness Around

Conclusion

Step 1: Identify, Accept, and Label Your Anxiety

Being sleepless, experiencing a constantly racing mind, constant tension, future projecting, and having a debilitating mindset are all different clues that show you are anxious. Experiencing all these elements takes a toll on you, which is why you MUST overcome anxiety.

The first basic step to overcoming anxiety is accepting your anxiousness as it happens. To understand the notion of accepting your anxiety as it happens, let us explore how to do that:

What happens when you constantly run away from a worry? You only escape it temporarily, but the worry continues to grow and makes your life miserable. This is the case with anxiety.

You cannot manage and eliminate anxiety from your life because you constantly avoid it, have never accepted your anxiety, or made peace with the fact that you are a victim of anxiety. Because you do not accept it, it becomes impossible to control your racing thoughts.

To overcome anxiety, the first thing you need to do is identify and accept your anxiety as it happens.

How to Identify Your Anxiety As It Happens

Whenever you feel anxious, tell yourself, *"I am nervous and anxious."* This simple confrontation will give you a little peace because it will help you accept the fact that you do have a problem.

Once you identify your condition, tell yourself, *"Although I am feeling anxious, I am working hard to triumph over my condition."* This second suggestion will instill some calmness into your mind because you know you do have a problem and you are working towards dealing with the problem.

How to Label Your State

Next, take a journal and pen, and label it *"My Anxiety Journal."* Write down the date and the day, and then pen down your thoughts in that journal. Explain how you feel, define your situation, and describe the various emotions you experience when you become anxious. This simple practice will help you realize you suffer from a condition that needs treatment.

Although, verbal acceptance of your state is indeed an effective way to accept your situation, having a written account of it helps you label your condition, and makes you see how bad it has made your life.

Make a point of journaling your daily encounters with anxiety and the steps you take to battle it. Doing this will help you understand your condition better, as well as how well you are doing in dealing with the situation.

Accept Your Anxiety: It does not define you

Once you have identified and labeled your state of anxiety, you need to execute another important step: understand that although you suffer from a condition that needs treatment, being anxious is not your destiny.

Suffering from anxiety does not mean you are mentally disabled, or you are a psycho; it simply means you have a problem that needs management, which is not a label you need to live with throughout your life.

To accept your anxiety and keep it from defining you, utter positive suggestions such as *"I am an anxiety victim, yes, but I am also a confident and amazing individual who is going to combat and overcome my issue."*

This simple practice will boost your self-esteem and help you see that you have the power to control and get rid of your problem, and you will do it.

Step 2: Accept Change Is Progressive and Your Today Does Not Define Your Tomorrow

Dealing with anxiety boils down to accepting your condition, state, and the various associated elements. After making peace with being an anxiety victim, and labeling your anxiety as it happens, the next step is to accept yet another related reality: *while you may not be able to do much about your condition right now, it does not mean your future is grim and all hope for an anxiety-free tomorrow is lost.* **Understand that curing anxiety is a long process, sometimes, a life-long process similar to battling drug abuse.**

After accepting your condition, you may, in your excitement, feel compelled to rush through the entire 'anxiety curing' process. You may focus too much on the anxiety triggering thoughts in attempts to coerce them out of your mind, only to realize that you exacerbate the problem instead of treating it.

To prevent this from happening, YOU MUST understand that curing anxiety is a process. It takes time to treat a condition you allowed to grow bigger and fiercer. Just as you cannot get rid of a life threatening disease in a day or two, while it is the first step, accepting your anxiousness does not automatically lead to its elimination from your life.

After you understand this important fact, the fact that overcoming anxiety is not something you can immediately gratify, understand that by taking directed action oriented steps today, you can create a better and anxiety free tomorrow. Which directed steps are we talking about?

Accept anxiety is curable

Overcoming anxiety takes time; however, because it takes time does not mean anxiety is not curable; it is. With time, patience, experience, trust, persistence, and faith in yourself, you will kick anxiety out of your life for good.

This honest revelation will help you realize that, like a long arduous journey, your problem has an end; and if you persistently work towards reaching that end, despite the many ups and downs you will experience as you circumnavigate the journey, when you finish the journey, anxiety will cease controlling the reigns of your life.

Stay calm when you have a panic attack

Once you understand that dealing with anxiety is a steady progressive process, apply the following technique to your anxiousness and panic attacks.

Whenever you experience a panic attack, sit in a quiet, calm room, and do not engage in anything at all. Usually, a full-blown anxiety attack lasts anywhere between 20 to 60 minutes.

When you experience one, understand that instantly overcoming it is not a possibility especially because you are just starting to rein in your anxiety; therefore, all you have to do while you become anxious is to remain calm and let the anxiety be.

However, to overcome the anxiety, make one small change to your regular mode of handling your situation: *instead of fretting when a panic attack strikes, try not to give it any importance.*

Understand that when you do not bar them from leaving, like clouds, thoughts come, flow in your mind, and leave. Therefore, do not pause on a thought or meditate upon it.

Let anxiety-activating thoughts slowly exit your mind as quickly as they enter it; this will ensure they stop wreaking much havoc on your mind. While this practice seems simple, it is highly effective. If you regularly implement this step, it is going to provide you relief from routine panic attacks.

One highly effective technique you can use is meditation.

So far so good! Before you forget, I want to invite you to leave an honest review of this book. Thank you!!!

Step 3: Make Changes and the Right Choices Right Now

After accepting your anxiety has no instant cure, you need to make yet another important acknowledgement: while it is impossible to instantaneously overcome anxiety, there is much you can do right now to rein your anxiety.

How to Presently Make Positive Changes

To cure your anxiety, you not only have to get rid of the negative and poisonous thoughts that plague you mind, you also need to do a lot.

Your anxiety arises from various elements, factors, and situations of your life; to overcome anxiety, you also need to change all those negative factors and conditions. For instance, if you are in the habit of self-medicating by consuming alcoholic or caffeinated beverages, smoke or indulge in sweet pleasures, or binge eat to drown your anxiety, you must stop doing this because while these actions and choices offer temporally relief, in the end, their results are negative. In fact, these factors increase your anxiety and strengthen it.

Studies have shown that alcoholic and caffeinated drinks, smoking, and increased sugar intake aggravates anxiety.

These and many other behaviors and actions are factors that reinforce and worsen your problem. Therefore, to improve your condition, make positive changes in your life and make the right healthy choices.

Some positive changes you can adopt include:

Identify Negative Behaviors That Increase Your Condition And Improve Them

Once you understand the effect of negative and unhealthy behaviors and practices on your life and anxiety, attempt to identify all negative practices and slowly change them into positive and healthy ones.

Here are some well-known negative practices that augment anxiousness and that need replacement with positive behaviors and exercises.

Negative habit 1: Devouring calorie rich foods

If you are in the habit of munching on calorie rich foods, be it snacks or desserts each time you feel depressed and nervous, it could be one reason why you cannot overcome your anxiousness. If this is you, here is how to replace this negative reward:

Positive replacement: Shift to healthy and nutritious foods

Instead of consuming a diet rich in trans-fats, artificial ingredients, sodium, processed sugar, and genetically modified foods, make room for healthy and nutritious foods. Healthy foods include lean meat cuts, fresh fruits, vegetables, milk, soy goods, nuts, and essential oils. Additionally, stay hydrated by drinking 10 to 12 glasses of clean water every day. Water calms your nerves and stabilizes your mood, which curbs anxiety.

Increase your consumption of foods rich in tryptophan, precursor of serotonin, a mood improving neurotransmitter. When serotonin levels in your body improve, you become calmer and peaceful, and can successfully fight anxiety. Tryptophan rich foods include turkey, bananas, cheese, oats, nuts, soy, chicken, sesame seeds, and peanut butter.

Negative habit 2: Smoking and heavy consumption of alcohol and caffeine

Studies show that [alcohol aggravates your anxiety](#) because it adversely affects levels of serotonin in your brain; when the serotonin levels in your brain and body decrease, you feel anxious.

Similarly, caffeine and tobacco negatively influence your anxiety, which is why, if you truly want to rid your life of anxiety, you must gradually cut back on your alcohol, cigarettes, and caffeine consumption and work towards completely eliminating these elements from your life for good.

Positive replacement: Use chewing gum, juices and nuts

When you feel anxious, your first instinct is to light up a cigarette, drink a bottle of white wine, or increase your caffeine intake; as a result, you become 'jitterier'. Instead of doing this, always carry with you a pack of sugar free chewing gum, a bowl of nuts, or a bottle of fresh juice.

Whenever you feel nervous and crave unhealthy foods, chew sugar free gum, munch on a handful of nuts, or sip a glass of fresh orange juice. This prevents you from leaning on alcohol, caffeine, or cigarettes to cure your condition and slowly helps you get rid of these unhealthy practices.

Negative practice 3: Sleeping less

If you are prone to anxiety, another unhealthy habit you are likely to practice is to sleep less and stay awake longer. Studies prove that [sleep deprivation results in significant brain dysfunctions](#) that cause anxiety and exacerbate your condition. Additionally, extreme insomnia can make you hallucinate and experience emotional and mental symptoms similar to those caused by paranoid schizophrenia.

Studies have shown that if you are sleep deprived, you often suffer from significant brain "dysfunctions" that can cause further anxiety. In fact, extreme sleep deprivation can cause hallucination and make you experience mental and emotional symptoms that mimic paranoid schizophrenia. Hence, to stop being a victim of anxiety, you MUST improve your sleeping habits.

Positive replacement: Sleep for six to eight hours

To reduce and manage your anxiety, ensure to sleep for six to eight hours. When you sleep properly and give your body sufficient time to rest, different neurotransmitters such as dopamine and serotonin responsible for calming your body start to stabilize, which decreases your levels of anxiety.

To sleep easily and ensure you get enough sleep, set a sleep schedule and stick to it. This disciplines your body to follow a sleep routine, and slowly helps you sleep on time.

Secondly, create a peaceful bedroom environment by switching off the lights and ensure your bedroom is quiet.

Thirdly, make sure your bed is comfortable.

You can drink lavender or chamomile tea an hour before you sleep. Both these teas soothe your strained nerves, curb anxiety, and help you sleep easily.

Practice these measures and soon, drifting off to sleep will not remain a challenge; when that happens, you will learn to manage your anxiety.

Negative practice 4: Being sedentary

There exists a strong association between anxiety and an inactive lifestyle; a study published in the Journal of Neuroscience recently reinforced this link. The research study detailed results of researchers working at the Princeton University as they studied the link between anxiety and exercise on mice.

The researchers studied the brain levels of two groups of mice: one group had exercise wheels in their cage so they could exercise, whereas the second group sat quietly in their cage.

The results showed that mice that were inactive had an increased inclination towards anxiety as compared to the active mice. The same effect takes place in humans; therefore, to get rid of your anxiousness, stop being inactive.

Positive replacement: Exercise regularly

Replace your inactive lifestyle with an active one, and make an effort to make room for exercise in your life, even if it is for a mere ten minutes. You can engage in yoga, swim, jog, Pilates, aerobics, or play any type of sport you enjoy.

The idea is to become active while having fun at the same time. Start with exercising for ten minutes daily and slowly add a minute or two to your fitness routine after two to three days until you exercise for 40 minutes every day.

Not only does regular exercise lower your stress and anxiety levels, it also boosts your self-esteem and confidence. Exercise boosts your serotonin levels, which in turn enhances your self-worth and poise. When you exercise daily, you successfully combat your anxiety and become more confident, self-assured, and peaceful.

Negative behavior 5: Negative thoughts

There is a very close relationship between your thoughts and your anxiety. If your mind is full of negative, unhealthy, and unconstructive thoughts, you will never get out of the anxiety whirlpool swirling around you because when you believe in something, you multiply similar thoughts.

Your thoughts flow to the universe and have the ability to attract similar people and opportunities towards you. When you feed your mind with anxiety inducing thoughts, your subconscious strengthens your condition and brings negative events towards you that further worsen your condition.

Hence, if you say things like *"I am incapable of improving"*, *"I am failure"* or your thoughts and suggestions contain negative words, your anxiety will continuously heighten. To uproot anxiety from your mind, you MUST become a positive thinker.

Positive replacement: Practice affirmations

To rid your mind of negative thoughts, regularly practice affirmations. Positive affirmations are healthy suggestions you inject into your mind to harness the full potential of your super-amazing subconscious mind.

When you tell yourself good things, your mind slowly accepts them and begins to form similar healthy thoughts that frame your positive mindset, which brings endless, amazing possibilities towards you. Moreover, you can use this approach to tell your mind that you have the power to battle your condition and emerge victorious in that battle.

To practice affirmations, sit for 10 to 15 minutes in a peaceful spot and suggest positive things to yourself. For instance, to get rid of anxiety, you could tell yourself, *"I am strong, confident, and in a complete calm state of mind"*, *"With each breath, I exhale anxiety and inhale confidence'*, or *"I love myself, which is why I spread happiness and positivity wherever I go."*

You can use these affirmations or create personal ones; when creating personal affirmations, ensure they contain positive words and focus on the present, which means that you should use the present tense in your suggestion because doing so will frame thoughts that attract opportunities in your present.

If your affirmations contain the future tense, you will produce thoughts that focus on improving your future and your present will forever remain unpleasant and undesirable. If you religiously practice affirmations daily, in a couple of weeks, your anxiety will greatly diminish.

Focus on making these positive replacements of the negative habits to your routine because this is imperative if you are dedicated to perform miracles on your anxiety as well as your confidence because when you feel less nervous, your self-confidence, and self-worth increases.

Step 4: Practice Visualization and Anchoring

Bringing peace to your body, mind, and life may seem monumental at this exact moment; however, this goal is obtainable if you employ the following neuro-linguistic programming (NLP) techniques.

Visualize a Peaceful You

Visualization is an effective and powerful NLP technique that rids your mind and body of anxiety and helps you acquire inner peace. It works like affirmations, on the principle that positive and beautiful thoughts attract beautiful outcomes and opportunities.

To practice this technique, sit somewhere quiet, close your eyes, and imagine being peaceful. Envision being super-relaxed and calm, and enjoying your life to its fullest. Visualize being confident, having no fears, and easily interacting with others. Add lots of details such as colors, background music, noises, characters and other details that breathe life into this visualization.

The idea is to make your imagination so strong that you feel as if it is actually happening. You can practice this technique for as long as you like, but a minimum of 15 minutes per day works best.

Visualization has two main effects on yourself and life. Firstly, it will make you feel good about yourself, which will enforce the belief you can become strong, anxiety-free and self-assured.

Secondly, when you think positive thoughts, your positive thoughts move out into the open world and attract good things towards you. Therefore, this technique has no downside, only benefits and amazing things to you.

Anchor Peace in Your Mind

The second NLP technique is similarly extremely useful and powerful. The anchoring technique anchors peace and tranquility in your mind via a simple gesture.

To exercise anchoring, first practice affirmations or visualization so your mind becomes tranquil. Once your mind achieves some peace and tranquility, think of a color you associate with peace; sky blue is a nice choice, but choose any color you deem peaceful.

Once you have your color, visualize being inside a blue circle full of peace and harmony (or your preferred color), and those emotions engulfing your body. When your visualization becomes clear and strong, tie it to a hand gesture. You could press your thumb and index finger, snap your fingers, or use any other gesture you like.

Next, think of something else for a while, then practice that hand gesture, and instantly think of that blue circle full of peace. Practice this step about five times and then make the hand gesture one last time. If you feel peace brimming inside you as soon as you make your hand gesture, then this antidote has worked.

Exercise anchoring for 15 to 20 minutes daily. Within three weeks, you shall command it and will become peaceful as soon as you practice the hand gesture anchored to peace.

Step 5: Be Mindful of Your Blessings, and the Present

The next step toward being anxiety free and unlocking inner peace, complete self-confidence, and poise is becoming mindful and aware of your blessings, your beautiful life, the present moment, and the qualities bestowed upon you.

Why is this important? Well, you cannot achieve harmony until you become happy with whom you are and content with all your life has to offer you. To acquire and unleash inner peace, become cognizant of your blessings and be grateful to the universe for them. When you thank the universe, you encourage it to be kinder to you.

How to Become Conscious of Your Present

How can you become more conscious of the present and all the blessings it holds? Here is how:

The past or future do not matter, only the present does

The first thing you need to do to become mindful is to realize the importance of the past. For a moment, think of any worry associated with your past or future. Now, feel its effect on your mind.

Does it make you feel perturbed and restless? Do you lose the calmness inside you as soon as that disturbing thought enters your mind? Write about that feeling in your anxiety journal and then read it aloud. This will help you understand the disastrous effect of being stuck in the past or future.

Your present is beautiful

Next, give yourself some time to calm down and think of something calming and beautiful associated with your present; this could be something such as the new friendship you formed with a lovely person a few weeks ago. Think of how amazing that person is and how wonderful they make you feel. This is a thought and event connected to your present.

Ruminate on this thought for a while, and then feel what this simple practice does to your mind. Write down your feelings in your journal and then read them aloud. Do you feel good when you think of something nice in the present moment? Does ruminating on the present make you feel alive and better? It should.

Exercise this simple practice and soon, you will stop living in the past or future. One important thing you must remember is that the idea is to focus on the happy and good things in your present, so you can acknowledge it.

There will be factors in your present that you will want to remove and those that upset you, but this is a part of life. If you highlight the pros instead of the cons, you will completely ignore the cons. When you stop giving the cons importance, their negative effects vanish.

Know your strengths and celebrate them

Being mindful of the good things in life involves being cognizant of your qualities and the amazing individual you are. One reason why anxiety has shattered your life is the self-hate you practice.

You constantly focus on your few weaknesses, which causes you to discredit all the wonderful qualities that scream for your attention. Because you are a self-hate practitioner, you are likely to indulge in negative self-talk, which further lowers your morale and stabs your self-esteem.

To get yourself out of this dark pit, start by loving and appreciating yourself. However, this may be a little challenging especially because you are accustomed to abusing yourself.

To change this habit, give yourself the gift of time and spend quality time alone. Make a healthy beverage, sit somewhere peaceful and nice, and take out your journal. Now, ponder on who you really are and focus on your strengths, achievements, and good qualities. It may take time to write down a few, but be persistent and you will reach there.

List down any qualities and strengths that come to your mind no matter how irrelevant it seems and write a little description alongside each quality.

For instance, if you write, *"I am helpful",* write why you think you have this quality and give a few reasons to support your theory. Because anxiety has made you doubtful of yourself, this little description will validate your strengths and make you understand that you are an amazing person in possession of some amazing qualities.

Once you are done, go through your list, and read them loudly. Go slow and let each word sink; this will help you remain in the present and keep your thoughts from drifting to the past or future. Make sure to practice once daily because it will open you up to the fact that you are a wonderful person who deserves self-love.

Be aware of your blessings

Your next task is to become fully conscious and aware of your blessings. To do that, here is a simple exercise.

Switch off your phone and television because they distract you from the present, and make you worry about what you do not have, and what you could have. Then, take your journal and write down any three things in your life that you feel make your life comfortable and better.

For instance, a pair of new slippers because they keep your feet clean and comfortable, your spouse because you have someone who loves and cares for you and listens to you, and healthy food in your fridge. Wow! You have three amazing blessings in your life, and you thought you were living a hopeless and terrible life.

Listing your blessing will help you realize what you were missing by disregarding your present. Make sure to exercise this helpful tactic daily. The more you do it, the more you will become mindful of your amazing present and fall in love with it. When you start to accept yourself, your life, and your present as they are, you stop bothering about what you do not have and slowly become peaceful.

Thank the universe

Once you identify your blessings, build thankful affirmations around them. For instance, you could say, *"I am thankful for the wonderful life I have,"* *"I am grateful to the universe for giving me a beautiful life"* or *"I love myself, my life, and this universe."*

These affirmations center on the fact that you love your present, and you are pleased with the universe. This beautiful act of gratitude grounds you in the present and helps you establish peace with the universe. When you become good friends with the universe, it starts to offer you with peace, tranquility, and amazing blessings.

Make gratitude and acceptance a regular part of your life because being grateful and accepting will eliminate anxiety, tension, and stress from your life.

Step 6: Practice Regular Meditation

Meditation is a brilliant practice that trains your mind to be conscious of the blessings you have, to get insight into your thoughts, and to understand yourself.

Meditation effectively gets rid of all negative conditions and elements in your life, including anxiety and negative thinking. In addition, it strengthens your ability to focus on the present, become mindful of it, and practice gratefulness to the universe. Thus, to eliminate anxiety from your life, meditation is something you must learn and exercise daily.

How to Meditate For Anxiety Relief

Here is how to meditate for anxiety relief:

Choose a quiet meditation spot

To start meditating, start with choosing a meditation spot. Select a calm area and make sure the area or spot is distraction free by removing items that may cause you to lose interest in your meditative practice.

Comfortably sit down for 2 minutes

Next, sit down in a comfortable position on the ground, on a cushion, on your yoga mat, or even on a chair if sitting on the ground is uncomfortable. Tell yourself the practice will only last for two minutes and you need to focus on it for that short time.

Be conscious of your breathing

Next, slowly focus on your breathing and become completely conscious of it. Although our breath is constant, we are seldom aware of it. When you become conscious of your breathing, you slowly calm your mind.

When your mind calms down, it exits a state of active thinking and enters a state of peacefulness. When your mind is in an active thinking mode, thoughts race in your head and you have little to no control over them. However, when you relax, you slow down the speed of the moving thoughts, which gives you enough time to spot negative thoughts and understand their effect. When you become cognizant of your breathing, you slowly unwind your mind and start to relax.

As you remain conscious of your breath, breathe naturally and do not increase or decrease the speed at which you breathe. With time and practice, you will automatically start breathing deeply because you will reach a calm state of mind. Also, realign your concentration on your breathing if your thoughts wander away to something else.

Focus on your breathing for two minutes and slowly add more time to this practice with each passing day. In about two weeks, you will be able to meditate for ten minutes. When that happens, and you feel you no longer become distracted when you meditate, start focusing on your thoughts, so you can easily discern between the negative and the positive ones, and kick the former out of your system.

With time, you will have better insight into who you are and how your mind works. To reach this point, meditate with deep conviction daily.

Step 7: Be Around Positive People and Spread Happiness Around

The last thing you need to do to cure anxiety is to eliminate negative people from your life, and spread kindness and happiness everywhere.

The people you spend time with have a direct impact on your thoughts and your mindset. If you spend time with positive people, they will encourage you, support, and motivate you to be better.

However, if your company comprises of negative people who lack inspiration or motivation to improve their life, they will cast their negative influence on you and make you feel negative about yourself too.

Therefore, you must identify all negative influences in your life and slowly filter them out. When you eliminate negative people from your life, their negative auras will not affect you, which will make it easier to focus on improving yourself.

Additionally, focus on all the positive and supportive people in your life, and spend quality time with them. They are your support system; they will help you acquire peace of mind by supporting you as you battle anxiety.

Lastly, become a conduit of happiness, kindness, and positivity. Spread these positive emotions and elements around you and help others in distress become happier and relaxed.

Because positive people helped you combat anxiety, it is your time to do the same for someone in need. When you are kind to others, you feel good about yourself, which consequently makes you peaceful.

Find out if any of your friends, family members, or colleagues are suffering from anxiety and offer to help them. You could also visit shelter homes and help people there. Look for ways to be helpful; you will easily come across many.

Make kindness a permanent part of your personality because kindness is a powerful element that battles negative, anxiety inducing thoughts.

Conclusion

You can successfully overcome anxiety and negativity if you implement each strategy discussed in this guide and stay true to your mission.

Above everything we have looked at and learnt, remember that overcoming anxiety to become a super positive person is a gradual process. The key idea is to form positive habits that support growth.

Thank you again for downloading this book!

I hope this book was able to help you gain some insight on what to do to overcome anxiety.

The next step is to put what you have learnt into practice.

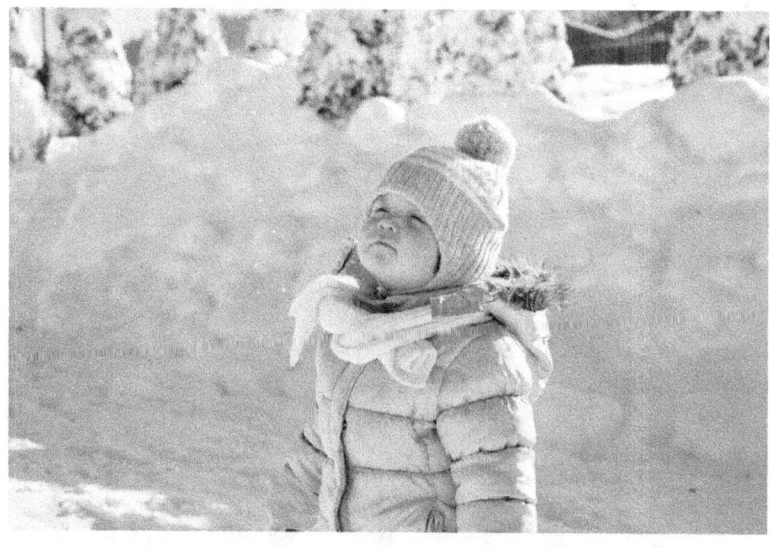

Finally, if you enjoyed this book, would you be kind enough to leave a review for this book on Amazon?

Thank you and good luck!

Anxiety

Free Yourself from Shyness, Constant Worry, and Trepidation

By: Sammy Parker

Understand The Root of Your Emotion, What's Causing Them, And Why. Take Charge of Your Life, Conquer Your Fear, And Find Relief From Acute and Chronic Stressors

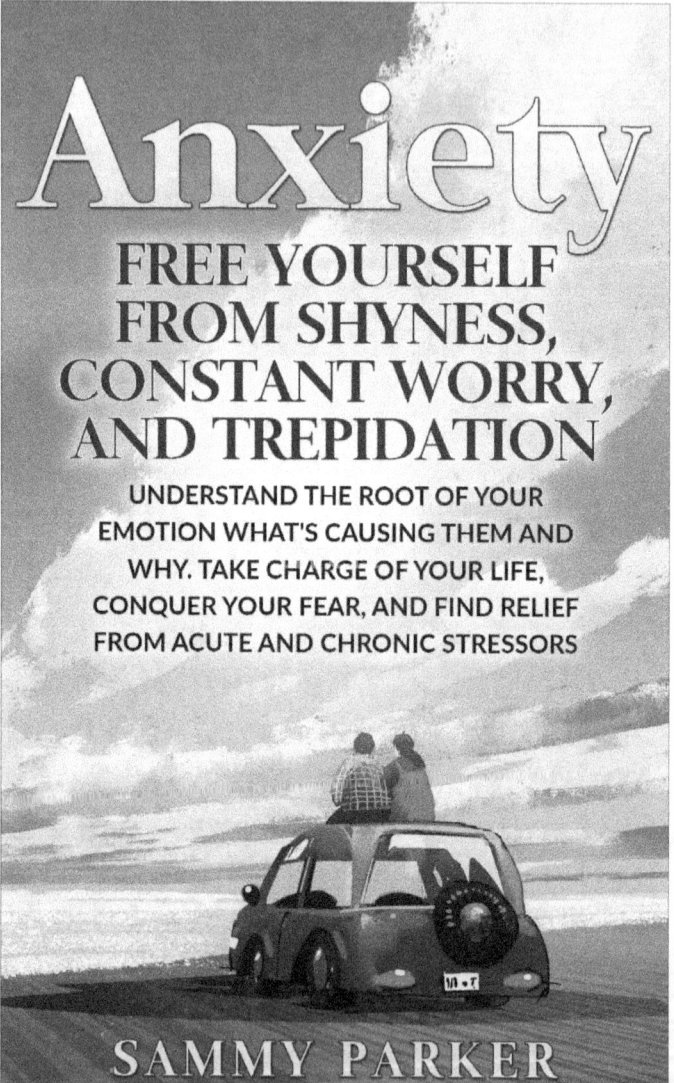

© Copyright 2014 by Sammy Parker - All rights reserved.

This document is geared towards providing exact and reliable information in regards to the topic and issue covered. The publication is sold with the idea that the publisher is not required to render accounting, officially permitted, or otherwise, qualified services. If advice is necessary, legal or professional, a practiced individual in the profession should be ordered.

- From a Declaration of Principles which was accepted and approved equally by a Committee of the American Bar Association and a Committee of Publishers and Associations.

In no way is it legal to reproduce, duplicate, or transmit any part of this document in either electronic means or in printed format. Recording of this publication is strictly prohibited and any storage of this document is not allowed unless with written permission from the publisher. All rights reserved.

The information provided herein is stated to be truthful and consistent, in that any liability, in terms of inattention or otherwise, by any usage or abuse of any policies, processes, or directions contained within is the solitary and utter responsibility of the recipient reader. Under no circumstances will any legal responsibility or blame be held against the publisher for any reparation, damages, or monetary loss due to the information herein, either directly or indirectly.

Respective authors own all copyrights not held by the publisher.

The information herein is offered for informational purposes solely, and is universal as so. The presentation of the information is without contract or any type of guarantee assurance.

The trademarks that are used are without any consent, and the publication of the trademark is without permission or backing by the trademark owner. All trademarks and brands within this book are for clarifying purposes only and are the owned by the owners themselves, not affiliated with this document.

Table of Contents

Introduction

Chapter 1: What is Anxiety?

Chapter 2: Common Types of Anxiety

Chapter 3: The Common Misconceptions

Chapter 4: Understanding the Root of Your Emotion, What's Causing Them, and Why

Chapter 5: Taking Charge of Your Life with Anxiety

Chapter 6: Conquering Your Fear

Chapter 7: Anxiety on Children

Conclusion

Introduction

For many people who are struggling with anxiety every year, living a normal life seems to be one of the most challenging things to do. There are treatments and medicines currently out there, but sometimes it is not enough to overcome this reoccurring and debilitating ailment. It is important to remember that millions of people worldwide suffer from anxiety and that you are not alone in this fight. What's more important is that there are professionals out there who can help you. However, it is imperative to know that there specific things you can do to help yourself first. The first thing that a person who suffers from anxiety has to do is learn how to live life carrying this condition. As easy as it sounds, it is the hardest part, as the natural response for a person from this incapacitating condition is to escape the issue completely.

In deciding how to live with Social Anxiety Disorder, running and hiding is not a real option – rather, it is not an option at all. If, you truly want to live, there is only one way to achieve that: you MUST make a plan for treating your disorder, and you MUST stick with your plan until you succeed. Of course, the first step is to obtain a diagnosis of your anxiety, but the fact that you are wondering how to live with Social Anxiety Disorder is a pretty good indication that you already know that you have it.

There are hundreds and thousands of websites and books available that talk about general anxiety disorder, anxiety attacks, symptoms, and consequences, but not a lot of them talk about how life truly is through the lens of an actual person suffering from anxiety.

I am a victim of anxiety myself. And I got to say that it's definitely one of the hardest experiences I had to deal with in my life and I don't wish it on anyone. School exams, riding a roller coaster, traveling alone, job interviews, meeting new people, crowded places...the list goes on and on. As you can imagine, I've had a lot of problems enjoying memorable events in my life the way any normal person would. Are you wondering why? That's because being shy, constant worry, and always fear for the worst were drowning my life, which prevented me from LIVING in the moment.

So obviously, on those events where I had anxiety, I felt so frantic, so frightened that I was convinced I was about to die at any moment. With that mindset, how could I possibly enjoy the actual moment itself? In other words, if I experience panic attacks after spending the whole day swimming at my dream beach, riding the plane, or watching a concert with a big crowd, all my future memories die together with the memories of trembling, fast heartbeats, lightheadedness, awful headaches, and nausea. That's not all; most of the time I also experience an awful feeling of dread of paralyzing fear.

Living with anxiety is absolutely not easy. I've had to meet more than a few doctors and it took me a long time to find a psychiatrist and a psychologist that helped and encouraged me to find tools within myself, which allowed me to deal with panic attacks and battle those awful fears. Luckily as well, I had the support of my friends and family around me to always guide and love me.

My battle with anxiety has been a long, tough journey, but right now I can say that I have successfully overcome it. And as I mentioned earlier, this is something I wouldn't wish on anyone – even on my worst enemy. And with this book, I will share with you how I battled my anxiety to live life without shyness, constant worry, and trepidation.

Chapter 1: What is Anxiety?

First of all, to fight the problem, the first thing you must do is to get to know the problem itself. Anxiety disorders are conditions that make a person develop intense distress and fear for both real and unreal reasons. Throughout the last century, anxiety has been categorized under the science of psychiatry as it was discovered that fear and apprehension could affect both psychological and physical functions of those who are stricken. It's shown in numerous symptoms categorized into physical tension, psychological anxiety, and panic attacks. In a lot of circumstances, the anxiety continues unceasingly even though the threat of the object is not there anymore.

By understanding exactly what anxiety is, it's going to be helpful if you also know the symptoms you are struggling with. It's common for a person to feel real fear and distress attended by nausea, chaotic thoughts, trouble breathing, and quivering. Fear of things, people, animals, or situations is called phobia and is known as a type of anxiety disorder. It's normally generated by a bad experience, which involves the feared event, people, animal, or anything for that matter. For example, fear of dogs can be triggered by a bad experience such as getting bitten by a dog. Obsession is also a form of anxiety disorders. Obsessions towards a person, thing, or events, can lead to an atypical failure of the state of mind, which convert rigorous obsession to compulsive actions.

A classic example of an anxiety disorder is when someone is provoked by an insistent threat or possibility of destruction or illness from either business or work; the unceasing experience continues to give you fear that can last for minutes, to hours, or even days. This is what known as the panic attack. In panic attacks, the emotional state of a person starts to influence the physical condition and physical signs such as apprehension, running out of breath, and fast heartbeat are felt by the troubled persons. There are cases that the anxiety could reach up to 6 months and becomes a lasting condition.

Furthermore, anxiety disorders could also influence kids whom, when stricken by insistent fears and worries, undergo abnormal functioning in their social relations and learning processes. They undergo psychological depression, lack of motivation, and even regress in their intellectual and social developments. The physical wellbeing can also be affected as most stricken children experience dysfunctions such as upset stomach, diarrhea, fast heart rate, high blood pressure, lack of breath, nausea, and a lot of other indicators. A lot of people eventually experience trouble sleeping which further deteriorates their condition.

There's nothing fun about dealing with anxiety, and those who are suffering from this disease would like to know what anxiety is and what can they do to stop it. Most of us have some type of anxiety. There are some aspects of our life that are out of control.

If you're going to define anxiety like this, you'll think that anxiety isn't a bad thing. In fact, it's a part of the physical response of our body for fight, flight, or freeze in a specific response. More so, the heart races, the body gets all sweaty, there's difficulty in breathing, you urinate more often, it's harder to swallow, or the mouth dries up. It's when your body gets ready for the hormone release known as adrenaline, which can help in coping with nerve-wracking events.

But when does anxiety get difficult?

Even though it's normal to feel anxious during different situations, this only becomes difficult when you worry unnecessarily. If you worry too much about things that you can't seem to understand, if the level of your anxiety is unbearable, or if you worry excessively that it restricts your sleep and obstruct your normal daily routines, then you possibly have what's known as the psychological anxiety.

Chapter 2: Common Types of Anxiety

Yes, there are different types of anxiety, to learn more about them. Anxiety disorders can be categorized into more specific types. Below are the most common types of anxiety and their symptoms that people experience.

Generalized Anxiety Disorder or GAD

Generalized Anxiety Disorder is a form of anxiety recognized by extreme long-standing anxiety and fear of nonspecific situations or events. People who suffer from GAD normally worry about all forms of problems. This could be their career, relationship, money, or health but can't identify how to control their fears. This fear is normally seen by others as something pointless and exaggerated. Most of the time, people who suffer from GAD get anxious over things that have little to nothing of a chance of happening. They could also feel worried all throughout the day for no obvious reason. This form of anxiety can also affect its victim physically. Few of the physical symptoms one may experience could be a sleeping problem, muscle pains, and constant fatigue.

Emotional Symptoms

- Continuous worries going on through the head

- Feeling uncontrollably anxious

- Disturbing thoughts about things you're worried about

- An incapacity to put up with uncertainty

- An inescapable feeling of uneasiness or fear

Behavioral Symptoms

- Incapability to relax, enjoy silence or be alone

- Trouble focusing or concentrating on things

- Feeling overwhelmed to do things

- Avoiding events that you feel anxious about

Physical Symptoms

- Feeling tension

- Sleeping problem because your mind won't stop working

- Feeling nervous, twitchy, or edgy

- Nausea, diarrhea, and other stomach problem

General Tips:

-Look at the things you worried about in a new perspective. The main symptom of generalized anxiety disorder is worrying too much. It is important to know what worrying can cause you as the beliefs you have in regards to worrying has a big role in triggering and sustaining this mental disorder.

- Know how to calm down quickly. A lot of people with this condition don't have any idea how they can soothe themselves quickly. But it is an easy method to learn, and it could make a radical difference in your anxiety.

-Be physically active. Exercising relieves tension, decreases stress hormones, increases feel-good chemicals like endorphins and serotonin, and changes the brain in ways, which make it less prone to anxiety.

- Have an anxiety-breaking standard of living. A healthy lifestyle has a huge role in keeping the GAD symptoms controlled. Along with regular

exercise, try these other lifestyle routines to fight worrying too much and chronic anxiety:

- Get enough sleep
- Limit the intake of caffeine
- Avoid nicotine and alcohol
- Have a healthy diet

-Practice relaxation techniques. Anxiety is not just a simple 'feeling.' It is the physical "fight or flight" reaction of the body to a detected threat. Your heart beats fast, you're running out of breath, you feel your muscle tensed up, and you feel dizzy. When you are relaxed, these things don't happen.

- Get in touch with others. Getting support from other people is important to overcome GAD. Actually, GAD only gets worse when you feel alone and hopeless.

Post-Traumatic Stress Disorder or PTSD

Post-traumatic Stress Disorder or PTSD is a form anxiety that's brought on from the past situation that continues to upset the person long after that event has happened. These could be severe cases, for example, if someone was burgled or attacked to very serious cases like rape, hostage situations, or a soldier who was involved in a war. PTSD involves getting flashbacks to that certain event and could lead to stress behavior when the situation is recollected by the mind.

PTSD affects everyone in a different way. While the signs and symptoms of this type of anxiety are most commonly developed after the actual traumatic event, it could take days, weeks, months, or even years before they show up. Here are the three main symptoms of PTSD:

- Getting flashbacks of what happened.

- Avoiding things, people, events, or anything that reminds you of the traumatic event.

- Problem sleeping, prickliness, a problem of focusing, feeling nervous, and easily alarmed.

General Tips:

- *Monitor your nervous system.* Knowing that you are able to change your arousal system and able to calm yourself down, you can directly challenge the sense of helplessness that's a common sign of this disorder.

- *Socialize with people.* Getting support and encouragement from people is important to your recovery. Having some people to connect with is very effective way to calm your nervous system.

- *Look after yourself.* The symptoms brought by PTSD can affect your body significantly, so it is important to look after yourself and develop healthy habits.

- *Be physically active.* By exercising, you will release endorphins that make you feel better. By moving your body, you will not make yourself feel unstuck.

Obsessive-Compulsive Disorder or OCD

Obsessive-Compulsive Disorder or OCD is a form anxiety that could be repetitive and irrational behavior. However, the sufferer eases their compulsive disorder by performing a particular pattern with persistence like obsessively checking their wallets, washing hands, checking the light switch, and persistently cleaning personal things.

Just because you're getting obsessive thoughts or do compulsive actions, doesn't mean that you have this problem. With OCD, these behaviors and thoughts lead to great grief, repetitive fidgety reactions, and affect your everyday life and relationships negatively.

Obsessive Thoughts

- Fear of being dirty

- Fear of hurting yourself or anyone

- Invasive sexually explicit or violent imagination

- Extreme focus on beliefs

- Fear of not having the things you need

- Making sure everything is perfect and in order

- Extreme beliefs in superstitions

<u>Compulsive Behaviors</u>

- Repeatedly checking everything

- Tapping, counting, repeating certain words over and over

- Cleaning or washing something for long period of time

- Placing everything in order for no particular reason

General Tips:

-Devote to self-care. The way you live your life plays a big role in the feelings you get; it could help you cope your anxiety and live your life better.

-Try to resist your OCD rituals. If you have OCD, there are a lot of ways to help yourself. One of the most prevailing tactics is to try to break the compulsive behaviors and habits that keep your obsessions going. The key is to break one habit at a time and be self-conscious that you are doing that compulsive behavior.

- Challenge your obsessive thoughts. Obsessive-compulsive disorder can make the brain get trapped on a specific anxiety-persuading thought.

Social Anxiety Disorder

Social Anxiety Disorder is the fear of public humiliation and the fear of being judged by those people around you. Examples of this are perhaps a fear of being too close to others or if the person has to perform in front of a crowd. This form of anxiety could have a serious effect on someone by becoming isolated and avoids showing up in the public reaching critical circumstances that make someone lose his normal life.

Just because you sometimes get anxious in social events, doesn't mean you have this condition. A lot of people are just naturally self-conscious or shy; here are some common symptoms of people with social anxiety disorder:

Emotional Symptoms

- Extreme anxiety and self-consciousness in all social events

- Strong worry that lasts for days, weeks, or even months before an upcoming event

- Too much fear of being seen or judged by others, especially by strangers

- Fear that you're going to embarrass yourself by doing certain things

Physical Symptoms

- Difficulty of breathing

- Getting nauseous or having upset stomach

- Having shaky voice and stuttering

- Fast heartbeat

- Sweating

- Fainting or dizziness

Behavioral Symptoms

- Trying to avoid social events

- Hiding and being quiet

- Not looking at the eyes when talking

General Tips:

-Challenge negative thoughts. Social anxiety sufferers have negative thoughts and beliefs that contribute to their anxiety. Challenging these negative thoughts is an effective way to reduce the symptoms of social anxiety disorder.

-Learn to control your breath. A lot of changes happen within the body when the person gets anxious and one of the biggest changes is breaking the

breathing pattern. So to calm yourself down, learn how to control your breathing.

-Face your fears. Rather than avoiding your fears, the best way to get rid of them is to face them.

-Modify your environment. Joining friendly social environments first instead of going to a raucous crowd is another useful way to tackle and overcome social anxiety.

-Improve your lifestyle. While lifestyle changes alone aren't enough to overcome a social phobia or social anxiety disorder, they can support your overall treatment progress.

Panic Disorder

Panic Disorder is a form of anxiety classified by short, unexpected attacks of severe fear and worry that causes breathing problems, nausea, and dizziness. Panic attacks could happen really fast, but could last for hours. Panic disorders at times happen after frightening experiences or persistent stress, but they could be spontaneous too. A panic attack can make a person to be pretty aware of any change in typical body function, which interprets it as a life-threatening disease. Furthermore, attacks make a sufferer assume more panic attacks could lead to radical behavioral changes so as to prevent these attacks.

Panic attacks normally strike when you are far from home, but they can occur wherever and whenever. The symptoms develop brusquely and normally reach a 10-minute peak. In most cases, panic attacks last for about 20 to 30 minutes, and hardly last over an hour. Below are the most common symptoms:

- Hyperventilation or trouble breathing

- Fast heartbeat

- Chest discomfort or pain

- Shaking or trembling

- Choking feeling

- Feeling detached from the surroundings

- Sweating

- Upset stomach or nausea

- Feeling light-headed, dizzy, or faint

- Numbness or tingling feeling

- Cold or hot flashes

- Fear of losing control or going insane

General Tips:

- *Avoid smoking and too much caffeine.* Smoking and consuming too much caffeine can aggravate panic attacks in those who are vulnerable. Because of this, it is wise to not consume cigarettes and drink coffee or any caffeinated drinks.

- *Learn breathing control.* Hyperventilation carries a lot of feelings that happen throughout a panic attack. Deep breathing, alternatively, can get rid of the symptoms of panic attack.

- *Perform relaxation methods.* When done frequently, activities like meditation, yoga, and advanced muscle relaxation fortify the relaxation response of the body.

Phobia

A Phobia is an extreme fear of an event, thing, or situation that makes a person have a panic attack or a strong reaction towards something. Phobias like fear of being in a high place or fear of certain animals are pretty common for a lot of people, but there are so much more phobias of objects that could be seen as pretty strange yet still cause a person to have unreasonable anxiety attacks. In general, most people suffer from a phobia and find it easy to avoid these situations, but those who face their phobia on different occasions change their behavior immediately and feel the need to avoid it.

The symptoms of a phobia can range from trivial feelings of worry and nervousness, to a serious panic attack. Normally, the closer you get to something that you're scared, the bigger the fear you feel.

Physical Signs and Symptoms

- Shortness of breathing

- Very fast heartbeat

- Chest tightness or pain

- Shaking or trembling

- Feeling lightheaded or dizzy

- A roiling stomach

- Prickly sensations

- Excessive sweating

Emotional Signs and Symptoms

- Overwhelming panic or anxiety

- Extreme need to get away

- Feeling disconnected from yourself

- Fear of losing control or going insane

- Feeling like you are passing out or dying

General Tips:

-Practice relaxation techniques. Take time to perform a deep breathing exercise regularly. This just doesn't help you to reduce general anxiety but offers you a way to calm you down in certain situations.

- Change your thought processes. This could be hard but is important to when beating anxiety. Most of the time, when we face a difficult situation, you amplify the bad aspects or fear about the result, which make you even more anxious.

Adult Separation Anxiety Disorder or ASAD

Adult Separation Anxiety Disorder is a form of anxiety that puts a person with feelings of irrational behavior or panic when they're far away from things, people, or places they are familiar with, in other words, the fear of getting out of comfort zone. Some examples include when people leave their home to go to another country or city which separates them from their loved ones. They find it hard to get used to their new surroundings, which leads to extreme or unsuitable behavior.

ASAD has been unrecognized as a diagnostic mental disorder until the late 1990s. The symptoms of ASAD are not very different from childhood separation anxiety and may include the following:

- Repeated extreme anxiety about something bad is going to happen to their loved ones

- Heightened worry about getting killed or getting involved in an accident

- Wanting to be alone

- Refusing to sleep alone

- Repeated nightmares about being far away from their loved ones

General Tips

-Join a support group. This will let you interact with other people who can experience the same thing as you. Knowing people who are in the same boat would be a big help.

-Find things that will distract you from negative thoughts. When you start to feel fretful and begin thinking negative thoughts, you'll just feel more anxious.

-Practice breathing methods to help calm you down. Breathing could be a nice way to calm yourself down when you feel anxious. Deep breathing is known to naturally relieve stress.

Hypochondria

Hypochondria condition is where a person is excessively worried about being sick. People that suffer from hypochondria are what we have known as hypochondriacs. They really think that something's wrong with their body and go to doctors habitually to get a diagnosis.

Hypochondriacs don't do this for attention, but rather, they're really worried and anxious about their health. For example, someone cut his or her skin accidentally. Someone told them that it's possible for it to get infected; they will then start to think that he's going to get an infection so he goes to see 3 different doctors just in one day for the reason that he is terrified of it. They might be struggling with hypochondria. Other than this, here are other symptoms a hypochondriac is experiencing:

- Fear of having a serious disease

- Fear that the small symptoms are signs of a serious condition

- A lot of physical condition that normally change throughout the time

- The disorder can:

    - Last for about 6 months

    - Lead to major grief

    - Inhibit with work and social life

- Other indications include:

    - Getting yourself checked frequently

    - Having multiple checkups on different doctors for the same issue

    - Asking for repeated tests for similar symptoms

    - Reading information regarding particular illnesses and their symptom

- o Changing healthcare providers often

- o Trying multiple herbal medications or other alternative cure

General Tips:

- *Accept that everyone will die as it is a part of life.* Death is a natural process of everyone's life. It will happen to everyone. When you accept this fact, then it gets easier for you to not think about your illness too much.

- *Stop Reading Symptoms Online.* Most hypochondriacs like diagnosing themselves online after reading symptoms from WebMD. Keep in mind that not because you feel symptoms that a cancer patient experience, it means you have it.

- *Don't bring yourself to emergency rooms right away.* When you find yourself getting ill, don't instantly go to the emergency room or consult your doctor, doing this will put more pressure on you.

- *Try to change the way you think.* Take advantage of subliminal messages or suggestion to change your point of view. When you do this, you will stop looking at everything you are experiencing as a symptom of a serious illness.

Body Dysmorphic Disorder

Body Dysmorphic Disorder is a mental condition characterized by a worry about a defect in the physical appearance of a person. The flaw is either imaginary or a minor physical abnormality exists. The concern normally leads to major distress or damage in social, career, or other important aspects of a person's life. However, don't get confused this condition with other mental disorder such as Anorexia Nervosa. Some of the most specific symptoms of Body Dysmorphic Disorder are the following:

- Thinking that a person with physical defect or abnormality in their looks makes them feel ugly

- Repeatedly checking self in the mirror

- Avoiding picture taking

- Thinking that people are looking at themselves in a negative way

- Spending too much money on beauty products

- Being very uncomfortable

- Comparing your appearance to other people

- Trying to avoid social situations

- Wearing too much makeup or clothing that will hide their look

General Tips:

- *Avoid looking at mirrors.* Try to stop looking at yourself as often as you do. This will stop reminding you what you don't like about yourself.

- *Have a healthy lifestyle.* Getting enough sleep, eat healthy food, and workout regularly. Being physically active builds a healthy body image can help you to attain your goals.

- *Stop comparing yourself to others.* Don't compare yourself to other people especially to people you see on the magazine cover. You have to know that most of them are photoshopped.

- *Keep in mind that nobody is perfect.* Everyone has their flaws and you have features that other people envy about you.

Agoraphobia

Agoraphobia, which literally means "fear of the marketplace" in Greek, is another type of anxiety condition. It is a disorder where a person feels strongly nervous about being stuck in certain situations or places where people gather from which it is not easy to find an escape.

Concert halls, movie theaters, elevators, and public transport are some of the examples of problem places for agoraphobic individuals. They normally end up getting away from these situations or only go to certain places with people they know they'll be safe with. In serious cases, they might end up isolated, scared to go outside.

Agoraphobia can suddenly occur or develop over time, normally between people the ages of 18 and 35. It is a physical and emotional reaction to being placed into a particular situation that generates fear. Symptoms include the following:

- Strong feelings of dread, panic, horror, and terror.

- Knowing that the anxiety is exaggerated, but still can't fight it.

- Fast heartbeat, trembling, shortness of breathing and an irresistible urge to leave the situation

- Avoiding situations any way possible.

If left untreated, this condition tends to change in severity and can even vanish by itself. But if the illness stops you from socializing, working, or otherwise living your regular life, you must consult a doctor to ask for help

General Tips:

- *Perform Cognitive Behavioral Therapy or CBT.* This is strongly recommended for people that have agoraphobia to get rid of. This involves re-teaching people how to manage of their anxiety and body.

- *Challenge yourself.* Try to go to a certain situation that will trigger your fear but don't forget to do this with someone you trust.

- *Change your diet.* By changing your diet, you will improve yourself on the way you are going to react to certain situation.

- *- Avoid taking drugs and alcohol.* These items could considerably increase the symptoms of agoraphobia. It's analytically important for a person who has this to avoid using alcohol and drugs.

Again, I want to thank you for purchasing my book. If you've enjoyed reading this book, I would like to invite you to leave a review

Chapter 3: The Common Misconceptions

Anxiety attacks as could be explained scientifically nowadays by physiology and psychology, but still numerous people misinterpret these conditions, which make it hard for the sufferers to deal with it.

But you shouldn't use ignorance as an excuse; it is a chance to educate yourself. So read on below to know the misconceptions people throw on people struggling with anxiety...

Misconception #1: It's Possible to Avoid the Potential Triggers

A lot of people that suffer from anxiety have particular triggers that cause powerful feelings of panic attacks and anxiety. While a lot of people get anxious before a big event or getting in front of a big crowd, people that have anxiety normally gets scared being called on in a meeting or in a class. No matter what persuades a person's anxiety, it's not always easy to avoid or stop it— and telling the person that has anxiety makes it even worse most of the time.

Avoiding the triggers is not about preventing the person from entirely getting involved in life, in fact doing this will actually underpin the anxiety and leave the person feeling deserted and paralyzed when you culminate in a situation where avoidance is not a choice.

Misconception #2: People That Have Anxiety Must Drink To Calm Down

A lot of people that have anxiety are told by friends to just have some drinks to tone down. And yes, if the anxiety starts throughout the evening as you worry about the following day, it is very tempting to have some drinks. While it could help for the time being, its lasting effects can be dangerous. New research found that 13% of respondents who drank alcohol in the previous year had done so to tone down anxiety. The same research had found that people that have anxiety who self-medicate using drugs and alcohol were possible to worsen their condition.

It is generally alright to revel in a glass of wine while you're having a dinner, but alcohol must never be used as a solution to get rid of anxiety. Not only can it result in addiction, but it could also preclude people from pursuing professional help or developing healthy habits such as yoga, working out, and socializing.

Misconception #3: Anxiety Is Always Caused By a Specific Trauma

A traumatic experience is normally not the reason of social anxiety disorder or generalized anxiety. PTSD is a form of anxiety disorder, but those signs and symptoms are pretty different than what is experienced by those who have an anxiety condition that was embedded by brain chemistry and genetics.

People that have PTSD tend to experience anxiety that is directly associated with the traumatic experience they had in the past. Generalized anxiety disorder, on the other hand, is triggered by a combination of brain chemistry, genetics, and personality characters. People who suffer from generalized anxiety may feel very overwhelmed about speaking in public or talking to new people, even though they never had a very bad experience with either situation. So never think that those who have anxiety disorders are essentially experienced a traumatic experienced in the past.

Misconception #4: All Symptoms Are Nonphysical

When someone says he's feeling physically ill because of anxiety, you must believe it. Actually, some of the mostly known symptoms of anxiety disorder are physical and they are key indications that you have the disorder. Anxiety has a lot of physical side effects that the condition is often mistaken for physical disorders, which include tachycardia, asthma, heart problems, and ulcers. It is a rancorous cycle; since your anxiety goes up the moment you start struggling to breathe.

Misconception #5: The Person with Anxiety Can Easily "Calm Down" Or "Be Logical"

For many people who have anxiety, it's not a new thing for them to hear people tell them to be logical about the situation. People who struggle with anxiety know that a lot of their fears are illogical or irrational. What other people don't know is that people with anxiety are logically aware that a lot of their fears don't have a real basis, but they can't control their mind and body on reacting to certain things.

It is also a big part of why anxiety can be very frustrating and hard to explain to a person who doesn't have it. So when a person is having a problem with breathing and trying to keep it together, the last thing they want is to hear from someone that they should calm down and think rationally. For the most parts, these words could be very contemptuous and pompous.

Misconception #6: There's Nothing You Can Do to Stop an Anxiety Attack

Frivolously telling a person with anxiety to "calm down" is not helpful — but it does not mean that you can't do anything to help a person with this condition. If you know someone who suffers from anxiety, you can help them by asking them if they think you can do something for them to make them feel better when an anxiety attack happens. But, generally, some useful anxiety attack coping strategies include things that will distract them from the things that trigger the anxiety. Tell them to take a deep breath and even better, breath together with them.

Misconception #7: People That Have Anxiety Are Just Unreasonable and Illogical

As mentioned earlier, those who have anxiety generally know that a lot of their fears are illogical — and chances are, they tell themselves about it over and over. People with anxiety can't easily control their thoughts no matter how much they try.

That's why support from people they love is important for people who have anxiety. When we educate ourselves about anxiety, we're in an infinitely better position to help a loved one who is suffering — these supports could be in the form of encouragement or being on their side listening to what they feel.

Chapter 4: Understanding the Root of Your Emotion, What's Causing Them, and Why

At the first glimpse, it seems like different situations and events are the roots of having an anxiety. But let me clear it up for you... an anxiety attack can be triggered by a particular incident, sensation, sight, environment, smell, sound, or just an uneasy thought of an upcoming event. But none of those things are the REASON for anxiety; again they just trigger anxiety.

The ideas about the root of anxiety are not hardcore attestable. But therapists, scientists, and researchers show that the root of anxiety is divided into four main factors: hereditary, life experiences, personality, and brain chemistry.

HEREDITARY

First of all, your hereditary might be the thing to blame. Numerous research have found that the anxiety attacks could run thru families, which leads a lot of professionals to believe that the trait exists in the human genome. On the other hand, researches have done tests on identical twins revealing that there are cases where one twin will have anxiety conditions, while the other one will not. Another way where anxiety attacks can be hereditary is through an excessive cautious view on the world passed down by the patient's parents.

There are scientists that are studying family genetics as a root of anxiety. In two identical twins, when one of the siblings develops an anxiety condition, there's a highly likelihood of a chance that the other sibling is also going to have it as well. Moreover, there are studies that show that there's a bigger chance for a child will have anxiety if his parents have it.

LIFE EXPERIENCES

As a root of anxiety, psychotherapists generally believe that previous fearful experiences stuck in the subconscious mind initiate a person to react excessively to a common event or situation that other people can deal with without fear. A lot of researchers come to an agreement that root of anxiety is entrenched in violence, stress, poverty, or long-term or early abuse. When a person initially experiences panic attack is, a strong inscription is stuck on the mind of the person. This creates a cycle of anxiety in which the person cultivates a fear of having another attack.

PERSONALITY FACTORS

The type of personality a person has is a rather controversial factor, but a lot of experts agree that some type of characteristics seems to be associated with anxiety-related problems. A study shows that those who have certain personality traits are more likely to experience anxiety. For example, kids that are perfectionists, easily rattled, inhibited, timid, have low self-esteem, or very controlling, at times develop anxiety during childhood, adolescence, or adulthood. These traits are typically competitive and determined, with a propensity to disregard indications of stress. But it has also been discovered that such people can change their behavior, therefore, lessen the problems that they formerly experienced.

BRAIN CHEMISTRY

Some experts associate the root of anxiety to the brain's biochemical imbalance. A biochemical root of anxiety includes deregulation of neurotransmitters and chemicals such as noradrenaline, dopamine, serotonin, as well as GABA. This root of anxiety is possibly the most popular theory since symptoms could be calmed through medication. But this root of anxiety is still in high debate as there is no way to define if the person would have gotten relieved without using medication. For example, what you eat and how you move your body physically right now affects your brain chemistry and can chance the intensity and power of your next possible anxiety attack.

As you can see, there are a lot of possible roots of anxiety attacks, most of which are totally uncontrollable. The good thing is that it's not set in stone. What you have to realize is that you don't have anything to feel sorry about having this. You didn't ask to have it.

Chapter 5: Taking Charge of Your Life with Anxiety

Most of us now live in an anxious world. Whether you are worrying about how your work performances are, your diet, the welfare of your kids, or anything the keeps your mind working nonstop, our busy lives give us a lot of chance to fuss about what's going to happen for the next days, weeks, months, or years. Though as mentioned earlier that anxiety is a fairly normal occurrence, if it's stopping you to live a normal life as you used to, it might be the right time to start some coping strategies to get back on the right track and take charge of your life.

Take Time to Meditate

Because anxieties are normally tied to worrying about what's going to happen in the future, one of the simplest and fastest ways to keep them at pace is by focusing on what's going on the present instead. Taking a few minutes of your time meditating quietly could be a big help to sway away your apprehensions and to understand the causes of your worries. For most professional yogis, the breathing pattern and the way the mind works are connected. It is important to stop anything you do for a moment and focus on breathing to let the mind settle naturally. You can compare this phenomenon to a glass of orange juice that has lots of pulp in it; when you stir the juice, it will get cloudy in color, but if you just let it sit like that, the pulp settles in its position and the liquid gets a lot clearer – this is how anxiety works in our brain.

If you're experiencing anxiety as continues problem, then you can possibly manage it by performing meditation regularly. Take a few minutes a day to sit down, make sure that you do this during the time of the day when you know you know that no one or nothing is going to interrupt you and you can focus your whole attention on breathing. The consciousness of your breathing is helping in slowing down your heart rate level and helps your body to get out of the panic mode. If you're a busy person and finding time to meditate is not an easy task, then try to add a bit more mindfulness to your day by focusing on anything you are doing, instead of letting your mind think of something that is out of the present. For example, if you are jogging, focus on the breeze of wind hitting your face. When you are reading a book, feel every word and imagine the voice of every character written on it. But being mindful of what you are doing at present, you are helping yourself hold back your anxious mind.

Learn to Manage Your Thoughts

Knowing how to control your internal dialogue and thoughts is going to help you fight anxiety problem. This is also effective if your anxiety roots from your thoughts or ideas towards certain things. Those who have dysfunctional thoughts towards the things they are afraid of having bigger possibilities for their higher brain centers to tell their lower brain centers to panic, which provokes a fight, flight, freeze, or fawn response . You must learn how to delve into your thoughts more tangible for it to stop controlling you. This technique also emboldens continuing exposure to that which is the root of the anxiety, which helps a person comprehend there's no point worrying or fretting about that certain thing.

It is also much recommended to learn basic relaxation methods as a way to deal with anxiety, which includes progressive muscle relaxation that involves relaxing and tensing muscles located in different parts of the body. This helps the person get to know his body better.

Perform Yoga

It is important to learn how to connect with the body when you are feeling worried or anxious. Performing yoga is a way to combine mindfulness and movement. Exercise balances the body hormones. Though any kind of physical movement can be beneficial in fighting anxiety disorder, the contemplative focus offered by yoga its less goal-oriented approach could be mainly helpful to calm am anxious mind. A lot of people struggled with anxiety report that this practice has helped them to turn things around and live life normally again.

Have a Stress-Management Plan

Lastly, preventing stress is the main key to deal with anxiety. It is extremely essential to take some of your time every day for yourself, even though it is just for a few minutes of to listen to music, read a book, ride the bike to the park, walk your dog, spend an hour in the bathtub, or just anything that will help you divert your attention to something else. You will feel back in control of your again life in no time!

The secret here is consistency. I know it is not easy, but help yourself even more; you are stronger than any anxiety. Make sure to be always occupied and productive. By this, you are helping yourself not to have time to think and worry about things that don't actually matter and just live your life in the present and actually enjoy it.

Chapter 6: Conquering Your Fear

Every person has their own fears no matter how brave they think they are. Some might deny it, but it's impossible for anyone not to have one. It could be a fear of being old, rejection, dying, having an illness, losing someone, or running out of money.

Anxiety is a common phenomenon that most people experience every now and then. Being able to know how to cope with anxious thought is the best way to overcome anxiety. Don't let anxiety define you. Below are some useful tips and information to help you conquer your fear which leads to anxiety...

Anxiety Trick Explained

The Anxiety Trick is behind chronic anxiety that a lot of people experience. Have you tried to fight your anxiety, just to get unsuccessful results, or perhaps make your condition even worse? Anxiety Trick is the reason for this. This is a deceitful ghost that follows you everywhere telling you what to feel towards certain things, people, or situations.

It's an awfully common manifestation, and people falsely blame themselves when this happens. Here is a more precise and useful way to know this frustrating condition.

Anxiety is when you get tricked into feeling strong fear without any danger.

If you have an anxiety condition, you will be afraid when there is no danger going around. Their struggle to protect yourself from fear brings you to a path of growing trouble. That is the anxiety trick.

But how does it happen? Why do you feel afraid, even if there is no danger? Learn below how you get tricked:

- If you're suffering from Panic Disorder, your mind makes you believe that you are going to die, go insane, or fly off the handle of yourself.

- If you're suffering from Social Phobia, your mind makes you believe that you will look awkward in front of people and you'll be totally humiliated in front of people and they don't like you.

- If you're suffering from a Specific Phobia, your mind makes you believe that there is something terrible going to happen if you get close to or you did something that you are afraid to do.

- If you're suffering from OCD, your mind makes you believe that you have triggered a dreadful disaster. You may fear that you will burn the house down because you left the oven turn on or that you are going to be late for work for tomorrow because you didn't set the alarm, while in fact, you have checked those things more than a few times already.

- If you're suffering from Generalized Anxiety Disorder, your mind makes you believe that it is necessary to worry about certain things otherwise, something bad is going to happen.

In other words: You experience distress, and you feel like if you don't do something about it, you will be in danger

What does our anxious self, do when we feel like we're in danger? We do the fight-or-flight-or-freeze response —If I look stronger than it, then I will fight it. If I look weaker than it but slower than me, I will run away quickly. But if I look weaker and slower than it, then I will just freeze and hope it that it does not notice me. That is how we normally react to danger.

When you're experiencing a panic attack, an obsessive thought, or a phobic encounter, you will impulsively think that it's a danger. You will then, of course, protect yourself and choose which one is the best among the three – the Fight, Flight, or Freeze.

How Can You Overcome This Trick?

The thing that makes anxiety so persistent is the fact that no matter how much you try to escape, divert, or compete from your anxious thoughts and feeling, it will always be turned against you and make your anxiety a more insistent part of you.

So for a lot of people, the more they try, the more it gets worse. They are just putting more fuel on fire. So of course, the best thing to do is to stop putting on more fuel on fire. And this is where the cognitive behavioral methods come to the picture. They're intended ways to let you practice deal with the symptoms, not to fight them, but instead, to become less sensitive to them. As you're starting to lose the symptoms of your anxiety using this practice, the anxiety itself will then slowly fade away.

In order to deactivate the Anxiety Trick, you have to progressively spend time with anxiety, so as to expose yourself to the feelings and ideas, and let them dwindle on its own over time.

Always remember that exposing yourself is practice with fear, and make sure to do nothing to avoid, fight, or get distracted from its throughout exposure.

It is important for us to face these tricks in order to overcome them. This will teach our brains to learn something new. This is known as "corrective learning." This could be tricky, though, since we could still face our fears but still avoid them. For example, you were invited to a party. Since you are socially anxious, you are afraid to go, but because you want to face your fears, you attended the party, but the thing is, you were quiet in the corner and avoided conversation the whole time.

A good way to unlearn these unreasonable fears is to deliberately and recurrently confront them. This might sound cliché, but again, help yourself by reminding yourselves that you're not in a danger of any sort, you just feel uncomfortable. And this discomfort is what makes you feel that way. Always keep tell yourself that, "If others can do it, then so do you."

Studies have shown that when you confront something you're afraid of – which is not really dangerous – over and over, your brain will then start to respond to it differently.

All in all, your brain your brain is you worst enemy when it comes to anxiety. Anxiety is your brain telling you the worst case scenarios and skipping the best parts. But always keep in mind that there is something you can do about it. You must teach your brain to think logically and realistically. Again, in order to do this, you have to learn to face then rather than avoid them any way possible.

Chapter 7: Anxiety on Children

Anxiety disorder on children is one of the most common complications that children experience. Although children are commonly exposed to anxiety conditions, a recent study shows that not a lot of children are given a proper care in connection with this matter, which leads to chronic anxiety conditions as they get old.

Anxiety disorders cause the child experience worry and fear, causing a problem to their normal lives. These conditions can continue even after the kid has grown up; that's why it's important for parents to classify the indications to make sure that the child gets essential help and assistance. Empirically, kids who have got treatment or therapy are more possibly to entirely recover, or struggle with lesser attacks of anxiety.

Children have a higher probability to suffer from anxiety disorder and post-traumatic stress disorder, but other types include acute stress disorder and generalized anxiety disorder. Most of the common triggers are events like moving to a new school or a new house and the parents' divorce, which causes them to worry and be apprehensive. If not paid attention to, the child is more likely to suffer from low self-confidence, and chances are, the kid is going to be socially inept and lose interests to go to school.

For parents, it's then important that can classify symptoms of anxiety disorders on your children. You must remember that anxiety is a common emotion experienced by kids, and it could be hard to differentiate between a normal anxiety level and one that's not normal. If not sufficiently recognized and treated, the way the child thinks, as well as his learning dispositions can be strictly affected.

Symptoms could be psychological and physical, which range from nausea, headaches, and chest pains to extreme fear and doubt. Shows of such emotions are possible to change over time. Eventually, harmful levels of anxiety could turn into more chronic health conditions. As soon as you notice any of the symptoms mentioned above, it's best to talk to your child and consult a doctor.

Just like on adults, there are a lot of roots for anxiety on children, and that's the reason why it's a condition that is not easy to diagnose. Even though it could be hard to determine if your kid suffers from anxiety attacks, it's advisable to understand their situation.

Common triggers of anxiety for children include being scared of the dark or being alone. Remember that anxiety disorders are curable, and there are a lot of professionals who take care of children in treating anxiety. These vary from cognitive and behavioral therapy to medication, as well as other alternative treatments.

Conclusion

It looks like no matter how much we try to avoid it, getting away from anxiety is such a difficult thing to do. Living with anxiety is a part of many people's lives, which makes what could have been a fun, unforgettable experience turn into one that's full of uneasy tension. If you allow it to persist, it could make serious roadblocks on your personal and professional life alike.

If you're living with anxiety, you'll have to face two choices, which are either to give in or give up, or find beneficial productive means to courageously stand your ground and accept this tough enemy in a way that decreases its influence on your life.

The being said, not every person deals with anxiety the same way. For example, most women needed to talk their anxiety away, while men may prefer to keep their pain and may look for a more physical method to relieve their nervous tension. Other factors that may play a significant role in both how you see the world and how you deal with the problems that are certain to stumble upon you are hormones and age.

It's important that you learn how to manage anxiety, especially that many things around us trigger it. Most scenarios in our life can trigger the start of an anxiety attack. Knowing how to manage an attack is one of the first effective steps to recognizing that anxiety is actually present.

Though very possible, it can be hard to learn to how to manage anxiety. Most of the time, it's useful to look for professional assistance to guide you. A doctor is able to help efficiently ease your anxiety by explaining further and suggest what kind of medications you need to overcome it. Expect for you to be prescribed with medications that are proven to effectively work on many patients in the past. However, they may come with side-effects that your doctor will also explain to you.

Again, when learning how to manage your anxiety, you'll come to realize that regardless of how serious your condition might be, it's possible for you to overcome it. The first step is to know what kind of anxiety you have, and then know how to empirically observe these fears. Trying to distract your mind and looking for an expert's would also be good initial steps.

Hopefully, you find this book helpful and will try to apply some of the strategies mentioned on when dealing with your anxiety. Please always keep in mind that anxiety is a common occurrence to people, and a bit anxiety is actually pretty healthy to have in particular situations. If anxiety is stopping to live a fun, normal life, however, then know that there are steps you can do to fight it.

Thank you again for downloading this book!

I hope this book was able to help you understand a very general guide to Anxiety. Though it is very detailed and contains a ton of valuable content, I hope this book will serve you well in recognizing the type of anxiety you have and the different strategies you can take to conquer this disorder.

The next step is to practice all that you have learned so far and put into action of all the tips, advice, and recommendations to ensure that you will beat this nuisance of an ailment.

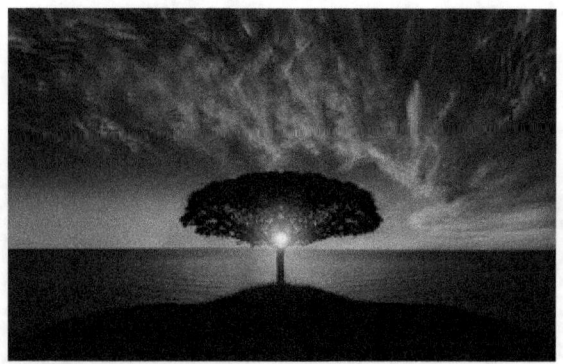

Finally, if you enjoyed this book, then I'd like to ask you for a favor, would you be kind enough to leave an honest review for this book on Amazon? It'd be greatly appreciated!

How to Analyze People: Using Human Psychology to Successfully Understand Anyone from Anyplace and Anywhere

Enhance your Social Skills, People Skills, Body Language, Relationships, Communication, Personality, and Nonverbal Cues

By Sammy Parker

Table of Contents

Introduction: Why is this Topic Important?

Chapter 1: How Knowing Body Language Helps you

Chapter 2: How to Improve Communication

Chapter 3: Building up your Charisma

Chapter 4: Making New Friends

Chapter 5: Strengthening Existing Relationships

Chapter 6: The dark side of human psychology – detecting liars, cheaters, and others alike

Conclusion

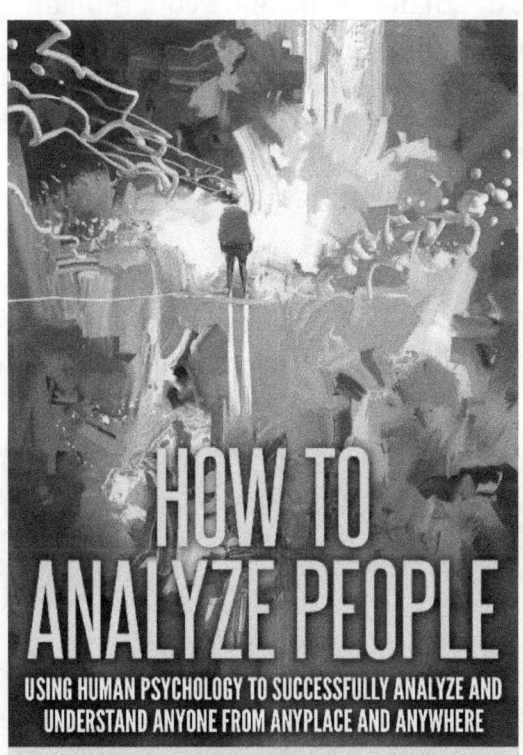

Introduction

I want to thank you and congratulate you for downloading the book, *"How to Analyze People and Use Psychology to Understand Anyone"*.

This book contains proven steps and strategies on how to get better at picking up the signals others are sending you, both in words and in nonverbal cues, to improve your interactions with people, in general.

This is an important topic because this type of communication is happening constantly, whether we are aware of it or not. It runs our interactions and rules our social lives, often without us even realizing it. Becoming aware of this aspect of existence will open up new doors to improving our relationships and ourselves with people, whether it be acquaintances or close friends and relatives.

In this Book, you will learn:

- **How to get a Better Idea of What People are Trying to Tell you:** People are not always upfront about their thoughts, feelings, and intentions. In fact, most of the time, they are portraying a lot of these at once without even knowing it. The people who have the highest success rates in dating, friendships, and any other area of life that involves human interaction, are aware of this hidden communication and how to use it to propel themselves forward. We will cover this topic in a later chapter.

- **How to Become more Charismatic:** It can be hard to know exactly what to say, especially when it comes to people you don't know very well or just met. For this reason, a lot of people struggle with having a lack of charisma, which hinders them in countless aspects of life. In this book, you will learn some proven ways to become more charismatic and draw people to you.

- **How to Talk to Strangers more Easily:** Talking to strangers is difficult when you aren't aware that you possess a high level of charisma and ability to read the body language of others. Meeting people you don't know will come naturally to you after you read the facts and strategies outlined in this book.

- **How to be a Better Communicator:** It's happened to all of us more than once. We have a message we feel is important to get across, we try to communicate it to someone near us, and they completely misinterpret what we said and it causes a huge confusion and sometimes arguments. This is often due to having inferior communication skills. After reading this book, this is a situation that will happen to you less and less frequently.

In essence, what you're about to read is a guide to yourself and others. You will find that the more you understand about your own motivations, fears, and abilities to communicate, the more you will be able to read and interact with other people. The two go hand in hand, and this guide will help you with both.

Thanks again for downloading this book, I hope you enjoy it!

© Copyright 2014 Sammy Parker - All rights reserved.

This document is geared towards providing exact and reliable information in regards to the topic and issue covered. The publication is sold with the idea that the publisher is not required to render accounting, officially permitted, or otherwise, qualified services. If advice is necessary, legal or professional, a practiced individual in the profession should be ordered.

From a Declaration of Principles which was accepted and approved equally by a Committee of the American Bar Association and a Committee of Publishers and Associations.

In no way is it legal to reproduce, duplicate, or transmit any part of this document in either electronic means or in printed format. Recording of this publication is strictly prohibited and any storage of this document is not allowed unless with written permission from the publisher. All rights reserved.

The information provided herein is stated to be truthful and consistent, in that any liability, in terms of inattention or otherwise, by any usage or abuse of any policies, processes, or directions contained within is the solitary and utter responsibility of the recipient reader. Under no circumstances will any legal responsibility or blame be held against the publisher for any reparation, damages, or monetary loss due to the information herein, either directly or indirectly.

Respective authors own all copyrights not held by the publisher.

The information herein is offered for informational purposes solely, and is universal as so. The presentation of the information is without contract or any type of guarantee assurance.

The trademarks that are used are without any consent, and the publication of the trademark is without permission or backing by the trademark owner. All trademarks and brands within this book are for clarifying purposes only and are the owned by the owners themselves, not affiliated with this document.

Chapter 1: How Knowing Body Language Helps You

We have all been in situations where we were either misunderstood by another person, misunderstood someone else, or even worse, a combination of the two. Some people are not very good at talking to strangers, making friends, or keeping existing relationships. A lot of these interpersonal misfortunes can be traced back to one very simple thing; being unaware of how to analyze others. This can lead to many headaches and rifts between others and us that do not have to be there. Luckily, there's hope for this.

Knowing how to Analyze Body Language will Help with:

- **Reading what is not Spoken:** Words are only a small portion of communication, and the rest comes across in our unspoken movements and gestures. Knowing how to analyze people will mean that you don't miss most of what is being communicated and know how to pay attention to it. This will help you become a master of communication.

- **Getting Messages Across more Clearly:** Once you understand how to read the unspoken cues of other people, you will better understand how to present yourself in ways that get across what you are trying to say. The people who are misinterpreted most often are usually not very aware of what their body language is saying. Sometimes, we say the exact opposite of what we mean or feel with our facial expressions or posture. Being aware of this side of things will make our thoughts and actions align.

- **Preventing Misunderstandings:** Being oblivious to the thoughts and feelings of others means that people see us as uncaring or perhaps even ignorant. This does not foster a healthy environment for healthy interactions or beneficial relationships. Taking it upon ourselves to learn about how to analyze the behavior of others and how to present ourselves more accurately means that communication, as a whole, becomes easier and we are presented with better opportunities throughout life.

These are just a few of the ways that body language can help you. It will also help you become more charismatic, since you will be more aware of your expressions than ever. Charisma is an important aspect of human life.

How Having Charisma Helps you with Life:

- **People Trust you More:** If you're a charismatic person, people tend to like you a lot more and a lot more often. This increases their level of trust in you meaning that they see you as someone they can rely on. This helps in personal situations as well as professional events or even interacting with people you have never met before. When you are a likeable person, doors open up where they never were before.

Old relationships can blossom in entirely new ways, you will find strangers opening up to you with an ease they never had before, and you will find it much easier to connect with people you just met, increasing opportunities.

- **It Helps you Stand Out Professionally:** The job market can be a competitive place, especially when you know that 10 other people are applying the same job as you. So, how do you stand out at an interview? By having unbeatable charisma. Work places get more and more competitive as time goes on, and the only way to stay relevant and up to date is to make sure that your personality is top notch.

This is a must if you want to gain great professional positions, keep the jobs, and also advance far in your professional life. This goes hand in hand with the trust that being charismatic brings, since bosses are more likely to promote people they trust.

- **Making Friends is Easier:** Having friends, especially a wide assortment of them, improves life vastly. Not only will you have access to more differing perspectives, interests, and hobbies, but you are opened up to a whole new world of personalities that you can look to for improving your own. You will also be better connected, meaning you have more people to rely on or to help you in hard times or with favors.

When you have a large friend group, you have a person to talk to about anything, no matter what subject arises, because of all of the different people you know and trust. This can only be possible when you are well aware of the body language of yourself and others.

Everyone wishes to be an intelligent and likeable person with a lot of influence. The only way this is possible is through knowing how to accurately read what others are trying to say and by getting a handle on the way we come across to others.

Chapter 2: How to Improve Communication

Now that we have identified the reasons why being aware of body language in ourselves and others is so important, we can get down to the basics of conversation. This isn't something that comes naturally to everyone, and most of us have to practice a lot before we become great at it. So, if you're starting out with getting comfortable talking to others, where do you begin?

- **Meet as Many People as Possible:** This can be a tough one, especially for people who are shy, but how can you improve your speaking abilities if you don't interact with many people? The first and most crucial step to being better at analyzing others and communicating with them effectively is putting yourself in more situations where you are interacting with new people. Over time, you will get better and better at reading their gestures, because being around other individuals will become so comfortable and natural. This may be hard at first, and you may find yourself distracted or overwhelmed by your surroundings, but this will improve the more you do it.

- **Don't be Afraid to Ask for Clarification:** Misunderstandings often happen because people are too shy to double check on something that someone said or did, and instead make assumptions. This habit helps no one and only treats tension where it doesn't have to exist. Whether you are talking to someone you know well and love, or a new person, if you aren't entirely sure what they meant by something they said, don't hesitate to ask! People are often more receptive to frank honesty than we think they will be, and showing this very human side of you creates rapport.

- **Get Feedback from Loved and Trusted Sources:** It's easy to see the qualities of others, but hard to see our own. For this reason, valuable insight can be gained from asking those close to us about our own traits that might be invisible or hard to see ourselves. Ask the three people around you who spend the most time with you on a daily basis what your great qualities are, and what aspects of yourself can use some work.

This will help you not only be more open and humble to the opinions of others, but learn how to improve your personality, which will bring you countless benefits in life. Don't forget to stay open for this exercise and remember not to get offended easily. If you think that a person you are asking would try to offend you with their answers, you should ask another source.

- **Start a Journal:** Becoming great at communicating with others starts in the way we talk to ourselves. Since many of us don't walk around having conversations aloud with ourselves, it can be hard to know exactly what those conversations look like. In fact, many times, they are subconscious and we know nothing about them!

The best way to get around this is to start a journal and write in it every single day. Even if you don't know what to say at first, you will figure it out quickly. This offers you a peek into the stream of your own mind, and once you get to know your own thoughts better, you will become better with interacting with others.

This is because, when becoming aware of our own stream of thoughts, they cannot distract us as much when we interact with other people. This is one problem that occurs a lot and gets in the way of communication.

- **Talk to Strangers more Often:** What is the best way to get better at talking to people? By talking to people, of course. You may be telling yourself that you "don't know how" or feel intimidated at the prospect, if you're the shy type, but this is one surefire way to get great at it.

If you aren't used to this, it may be a bit scary at first, but you will quickly learn that people are nothing to fear and are often a lot nicer than we think they would be. The more you practice speaking around strangers, the more comfortable you will become and you will eventually wonder why you held back from it for so long.

- **Join an Internet Forum:** This may sound like the opposite of communication to some, but starting conversations (and often, friendships) online is a great way to improve your speaking and ability to articulate your thoughts. No matter what your interest is, there is probably a forum for it, filled with people who are just as excited as you are about the subject.

This is a great way to get conversation flowing naturally with people you don't know. Here, you will encounter new questions and ideas, and in formulating your answers, you will discover that your ability to express yourself gets stronger and stronger, and not just on the internet.

- **Get Over the Fear of Looking like a Fool:** One of the biggest reasons we either hold back from talking to others or we filter ourselves in conversation is that we are afraid of how we will look to others. Where we are going wrong with this line of reasoning is that this type of withholding and hesitation is what creates the awkward tension that we all fear and try to avoid so much.

People who have been influential or seen as cool or confident people are always the ones who don't worry too much about what others think. This gives them a confident aura that others are inspired from, since it is quite rare. Keep in mind that everyone feels insecure sometimes and that there is nothing wrong with being nervous. Even when you are afraid, make yourself get out there and talk to people anyway.

Chapter 3: Building up your Charisma

It seems, at times, like charisma is something that you are either born with or not, but all people are actually capable of creating and improving their own charisma. Regardless of what your personality is like now, there are specific qualities you can become aware of and use with your behaviors that will likely make you more influential, trustworthy, and all around likeable. Here is some basic information about how to build up your charisma.

It's Learned, not Inherent in Humans:

When we meet someone we like, we can rarely explain exactly what it is about him or her that draws us in so much. This means that they possess charisma. You can also learn how to be charismatic, and it's easier than you may think. It involves a few small changes to the way you behave. This quality is all about the things you say and the actions you partake in, rather than your deeper qualities. Your nonverbal cues, subconscious attitudes, physical motions, and the respect you have for other people are all involved with your level or charisma and the steps you will take to improve it.

Although this is a simple process, it does take some bravery on your part. Building up your charisma is an event that will require a close look at your actions. This often leads to seeing things you don't particularly like, but it's important not to get hung up on that, since it happens to everyone who becomes self-aware.

If you know how to check your expectations instead of getting stuck on them, you will be able to see which behaviors of yours need to be changed. Keep in mind that you don't need to fundamentally change everything about your core self, only the way those around you will perceive you by tweaking your outward expressions. Here are some real, actionable steps for gaining and keeping charisma:

Learn how to be Present:

This is one of, if not the most crucial factor in building charisma, along with knowing how to exude confidence. Being present means that you know how to engage with other people in a real way. In essence, you are showing the individual you are interacting with that they have your focus.

- **Be Aware of How you Come Across to Other People:** When someone isn't confident, they can often come across as someone who doesn't have any interest in other people, even when the opposite is true. Without knowing how to be present for others in conversation, you could come across as arrogant or uncaring. Neither of these extremes is something to hope for. Being present for others shows them that they are worth your time and that you care to hear them out. Nothing works better for building respect and trust than this.

- **It's about Helping Others Feel Good about Themselves:** Some people may think of charisma and automatically have ideas of seeming awesome and confident in the eyes of other people, but the true secret to it involves more than this. Charisma is not about showcasing your greatness to the world, but about knowing how to make another feel great about them. This means that they feel important, worthwhile, and leave a conversation with you feeling better about life and their own worth than they did prior to the interaction.

- **Know What People Like to Discuss:** An inescapable fact about humans is that we enjoy speaking about the subject we are most familiar with; ourselves. When you like someone or find them charismatic or magnetic, it's usually because they allow you to talk about your interests and be yourself. Stay optimistic, turn your ego off, and be present for people when they are speaking to you. It can truly be as simple as this.

- **Find Ways to Stay Intrigued and Focused:** Give your utmost focus to everything that the other is saying, imagining that you are focusing on a book or movie and that they are the most important character, if this helps you. A lot of people talk to others while just focusing on what they are going to say next, without truly listening. This comes across in interactions and is a huge turnoff. While this may seem like you are truly engaging in the conversation, you aren't, and it doesn't seem as though you are listening when you do this.

Of course, this involves a balance of listening and speaking. It's not good to simply sit and be a listening ear for everyone without getting the same favor in return. Being aware of how to express yourself and speak to others in a way that exudes confidence is equally important to listening.

Increase your Level of Personal Confidence:

Learning how to become confident will give you a gigantic advantage when you decide to undertake the journey to developing charisma, but this is easier said than done. If it were as simple as deciding to have confidence, everyone would do it, and it wouldn't even be a noteworthy quality. You shouldn't want to come across as arrogant or self-absorbed, but it's equally negative to seem scared or timid in social situations. What it all relies on is your own level of comfort with yourself.

- **Confidence begins with the Physical** Staying active and in shape, wearing items that make you feel nice about yourself, and focusing on conversation topics that you can contribute to will make you feel more confident about yourself.

- **Don't Fear not Knowing about Certain Topics:** This doesn't mean that you should only speak about things you are an expert in, however. It's perfectly possible to stay on an open level with people and show them that you are interested and curious while still staying confident and assertive. A lot of people get frozen up when we find ourselves in a talk that we aren't knowledgeable about, which makes us defensive and oftentimes, awkward. We may shift to a position of trying to hide our own lack of knowledge, when simply being comfortable with our ignorance would come across as way more likeable and relatable to others.

- **Maintain an Open and Curious Demeanor:** If you learn how to switch, at will, from this mode of defense to a mode of openness and curiosity, you will come across as a confident person who is okay with the fact that they aren't knowledgeable about a certain subject. In addition to this, staying in a curious frame of mind will help you stay present, which we mentioned the importance of earlier. You won't be tuning out of the conversation or rehearsing what you will say next, you will seem truly present for the other person.

- **Find a Reason to Live:** When someone has charisma and confidence, their lives have a purpose. Not having a driving force or mission in life is something that is visible and noticeable to others, and it isn't a very attractive quality to be missing this essential characteristic. This doesn't mean that you have to enthusiastically rave about your passion at every chance you get, but you must be aware of and confident about the fact that you are alive for a reason.

- **Focus your Energies:** Select a goal, cause, or vision to become passionate about and life. Most individuals go through life searching for a reason to live or a cause to truly put their faith in. You must embody your passion so intensely that it is noticeable to others.

- **Fake it till you Make it:** Believe in yourself in every situation and show that you are not bothered by the doubts that overtake most others. Pretend like you know where you are going and why, even if you aren't completely certain. This helps a lot with developing confidence, over time. Even when you aren't sure where you are headed, you should appear to be aware.

- **Pretend it's a Movie:** As soon as a certain scenario starts playing out, pretend to be aware of exactly what your next lines are.

- **Forget Mistakes as Soon as Possible:** Everyone has times when we say or do something and feel, later, that it was the dumb thing to say or do. Do yourself a favor and banish those moments from your memory.

When those situations occur and you stop to ruminate on what just happened, the way you appear to others changes immediately. You start to hesitate and others can notice this.

Being confident means that you are okay with what type of person you are and the things you do, regardless of what this specifically entails. People are drawn to people who have confidence, regardless of what their other traits are like. Once you master the art of confidence, charisma is the next logical step.

Learn Conversation Basics:

People who have charisma are good at talking to others. They are aware of the best ways to begin conversations, keep them interesting, and hold the attention of others, always making them feel comfortable. If you aren't aware of how to communicate with those around you, it's an inescapable fact that you must practice this. Sure, it won't be easy, at first, but being brave and getting away from the self-doubting personality traits will hold many benefits, in the end.

- **Learn to Stop Avoiding Discomfort:** Most people avoid uncomfortable situations like the plague, which is why charismatic people, who aren't paralyzed by the fear of looking stupid or saying the wrong thing, stand out so much. Get over the fear of uncomfortable situations and put yourself out there to develop charisma.

If you are unaware of how to begin conversations, don't be afraid to use your creativity to come up with ideas. Firstly, you can muse to yourself about which topic you would prefer to discuss and which you would not. If it so happens that there are topics that you want to avoid, it's probably safe to assume that many others would as well. Keep in mind that it's usually simpler and easier to start a conversation by simply being nice instead of trying to come across as smart.

- **Opt for Nice rather than Impressive:** Trying to seem impressive or highly intelligent can either come across as bragging or arrogant, or just intimidate others, which does nothing to improve charisma. In addition to this, being nice to others is one of the quickest ways to instantly boost your charisma levels. If you are having trouble thinking of a way to open a conversation or find yourself in a lull during the talk, just find a way to avoid silences that could be awkward. More often than not, people will appreciate the effort.

- **Meet People on the Same Level:** People who are great at conversation know exactly how to get others on their level. They do this by sharing personal stories or telling about experiences in their life that relate to what others say. This has to be done in an artful way that doesn't attempt to shift the focus of the talk over to you, but only makes the other person feel understood and related to.

- **Rely on Humor, but in a Smart Way:** Charismatic people are often funny, but they know how to do it and when to hold off. Don't be afraid to use the valuable tool of humor but keep in mind that the way you say things is often more important than what you are saying. If you are uncertain about whether a joke is appropriate, it's best to hold back. No one will even know about it and it's much safer than risking an awkward moment.

- **Be Interested Enough in Others to Ask them About Themselves:** Everyone wants ot feel as though they are being heard, and the best way to give them this feeling is to ask them interested questions. The individual who leads the inquiries is usually at the head of the business meeting. People who come up with intelligent questions always come across as smart, which improves their level or perceived charisma to other people around them.

While many people focus a lot on how their answers will come across, charisma often lies in the ability to know how to ask questions. Asking questions doesn't require special knowledge the way giving quality answers does, but the ones who ask the right questions are often the most likeable of all.

For an example of this phenomenon, envision the host of your favorite talk show. They are likely a very charismatic person, which is how they landed that job. Although they are so charming and likeable, they are usually doing nothing but inquiring about their guests, and come across as in control and highly likeable.

Being charismatic has more to do with caring about others than it does coming across as knowledgeable or impressive.

Get Better at Holding Eye Contact with Others:

As mentioned earlier in the book, most of communication has nothing to do with words, and eye contact is a perfect example of this. Quality eye contact has the ability to communicate far more than speech does. It can show that you care about the person speaking, that you are taking the time to listen, and that you respect the other person's individuality and rights as a person. If you can't stop looking away of averting your gaze, it could come across that you are not interested in them, even if this isn't true.

- **Find the Right Amount be Experimenting:** This is a tricky subject because too much eye contact can have negative consequences, while too little is also bad. To get past this conundrum you can practice keeping your eye contact for just a bit longer, next time you're talking to someone. How does this shift the communication? How does it change how the other reacts or how you feel about the conversation?

Keep in mind that there are countless chances to practice this method, including people who live with you or strangers out in public that you interact with. You can even try it with your waiter or the person sitting across from you on the train.

- **Try to Remember People's Eye Colors:** Eventually, you will figure out what works for you with holding eye contact and what is unnecessary. The way you initiate eye contact is equally important as the length of time you hold the gaze. If you don't know where you should begin and are afraid of coming across as strange, attempt to focus on the other person's eye color.

Make it a point to pay attention to the color of everyone's eyes that you interact with and turn this into a regular habit. This will come across as friendly, interested eye contact rather than the dreaded creepy kind we all wish to avoid.

Don't Forget to Use your Body to Express Yourself:

Magnetic, charismatic personalities are expressive in a number of ways. When you know how to use your entire body to enhance what you're saying or emphasize your feelings, it does a lot to improve your quality of communication. Nobody finds stiff people interesting, magnetic, or charismatic.

- **Don't Forget to Smile:** People who smile are far more likeable and approachable than people who appear uninterested or angry. If often only takes a few seconds of holding a smile to begin to genuinely feel happy, then the rest comes without effort. Be someone that people feel comfortable approaching by smiling instead of appearing neutral or negative.

- **Observe Others First:** If you don't know where to begin with expressing yourself more often physically, you can begin by paying more attention to those around you, including animals. Think of the most physically expressive people you know who captivate an entire room with their gestures, or your pet dog when he gets excited to see you after a long day at work.

People like to be around others, as well as pets, who have a wide range or gestures that are highly expressive. This doesn't mean you need to be over the top with it or fake, but physical gestures that correspond with events that are happening and are relevant to the situation at hand are appealing and winning. They do a lot to increase your charisma.

- **Stay Aware of Negative Physical Expressions, too:** While focusing more on your physical gestures, it's important to be aware of what can come across as negative, in this regard. To take an example, nodding your head is a positive gesture to show a person that you are paying attention to what they are saying, but dong this too often can look awkward, wrong, and out of place. This can be a lot worse than not moving whatsoever.

Going over the top with your gestures can show to the other that you are attempting to come across a certain way and trying to make up for a lack of something. This means that they won't feel validated or safe around you anymore. Since individuals can sense your expressions, even the tiniest ones, learning to be aware of them is a great benefit to you.

If you are uncertain about what gestures you might do that come across as negative or awkward, you can ask a close and trusted loved one for advice. Remember that this might not be pleasant to hear, but you can never improve if you aren't aware of what areas you need to work on.

- **Stay Aware of your Gestures and Body Language:** Similar to actors learning to embody a character they are portraying, you should learn to get into a state of being that helps you stay conscious of how you are behaving. This can be something as simple as focusing on your breathing or simply feeling your body parts. Learn to realize when you are slouching or coming across in a negative way to others.

Learn how to Mirror Others in Conversation:

Humans are automatically drawn to others who have something in common with them, whether they are aware of it or not. Learning how to mirror the qualities of others is a quick and simple way to have charisma immediately. Make it a point to reflect back a person's level of energy or mannerisms and the effect it as will be noticeable right away.

- **It's not about Constantly Agreeing:** Mirroring doesn't mean you are trying to be exactly like the other person or need to agree with them on absolutely everything, but that you are meeting them on their level. With people who get along well or are great friends, this happens unconsciously, but it can be consciously engineered to increase charisma.

- **Emulate Charismatic Qualities in Other People:** Knowing how to observe and learn from others is a huge part of being charismatic. If you want to master this skill, the first place you should look is to people you find highly charismatic. This does not mean attempting to steal another person's personality or directly copying everything they do, but instead it means becoming aware of their secrets and what makes them great, testing them out for yourself and seeing what fits you.

- **Discover your Own Personal Methods:** The idea is experimenting plenty until you find the right methods that work for you, and this often involves borrowing methods from others that you respect. There is no "one size fits all" method, when it comes to anything. We can only look to experts and hope to learn from them by adjusting their ideas to our own lives and personalities until we find a good fit.

- **Observe Performers or Famous People:** You can find a lot of valuable tips on charisma by looking to Hollywood stars or anywhere else that you notice people with a lot of charisma. Pay attention to how they walk or speak. It's true that some of them might be arrogant or conceited, but this doesn't mean we can't learn from their charismatic or effective traits and use them for yourself. Learn how to borrow likeable traits from others and turn them into your own.

Everyone, including you, has the capability to become more charismatic and charming, meaning that others will like you more and more. The shifts you need to make and the adjustments that must be made for this to occur are not as huge or intimidating as you may think.

Simply become present for others, develop confidence, and work on mastering your physical gestures, over time, and observe the way others start reacting to you. Keep in mind that this pursuit, like any other worthwhile undertaking, will not happen instantly, but instead will be a process. As long as you are taking small steps in the right direction, each day, you are doing great!

Chapter 4: Meeting New Friends

Humans are social creatures, which means that having friends is valuable for everyone, no matter who they are or what their life situation is. They are the people we can turn to when things go bad, or celebrate with when things are great. It's hard to make friends or keep them if you don't know how to read body language or present yourself in the correct ways.

A very common problem that people have socially is that they are uncertain about how to make new friends or build a group of friends. This can be due to a variety of factors.

People Might have Difficulty with Friendships because:

- **They have Recently Moved and Haven't had a Chance to Socialize Yet:** This is perhaps the most familiar issue people face when moving to a new city. The reason moving can be so intimidating is because you are leaving everyone you know to start over, and building social groups doesn't come quickly or easily.

- **Their Friendships have Fallen by the Wayside due to a Serious Relationship:** This is a sadly common phenomenon. People forget about their friend groups because their romantic interest takes up most of their time or attention.

- **Old Friendships have Withered Naturally:** Another reason that people may have a lack of friends in life is because their old relationships have tapered off due to factors out of their control. This could be their friends moving to new cities, getting busy with their careers or starting families. An extreme version of this can happen when all friendships are concentrated in one area that is no longer there, such as a class ending and people all moving away at the same time.

- **Growing Apart from Old Friends and Wishing for New Ones:** Sometimes you simply grow out of friendships and would rather seek out relationships with new people who fit better with you. This can cause an awkward overlap where your social life is strangely empty.

- **Shifting from Preferring Solitude to Wishing for Friends:** People could feel a strong desire for friends in their life if they used to be the type who was a bit of a loner and have suddenly changed to someone who prefers to be around people and make friends.

- **Shyness or Fear of Speaking to People:** Obviously, a lack of friendships can result from someone being shy or not knowing how to approach others. Some people may be entirely unaware of how to talk to others and, as a result, have no social life.

- **Abrupt and Intense Life Changes:** When people make huge shifts in their habits or behavior, such as quitting drinking or even drastic eating habit changes, this can cause a shift in their social circle, since they may not fit in as well with their old one anymore.

Now that we have identified some of the common reasons people may be noticing a lack of friendships in their life, we will go over some methods for gaining new friendships. First we'll go over basics and then get into some more complex principles and attitudes that are crucial to the process of making friends. You will notice that people who seem to be natural at making new friends already do the stuff on the list.

How to Make New Friends:

Here are the easiest and simplest steps to building friendships. Some of them may seem obvious or simplistic, but each point can hold a lot of material. If you're someone who struggles with social life, in general, you might come across at least one of these.

- **Discover some Potential Friendships:** In order to find some new friends, you have to discover possibilities for who this could be. This can involve either looking to your existing contacts for potentials. Obviously, this doesn't work so well if you have just moved somewhere new and haven't met anyone yet, but usually people already have the makings of a friend group around them without even realizing it.

This doesn't mean you have to force yourself to go out on the town and talk to every stranger you see. You may find it better to look to existing people in your life and depending bonds with them rather than starting completely from scratch in building friendships. There may even be a few people you know already who are great candidates.

This could be acquaintance you get along with but don't see often. People you work with or go to school with and have an easy time talking to. Friends of family members or acquaintances. This could also be people you used to know well and have fallen out of contact with. Looking for ways to get the most out of your existing connections can be very helpful, but sometimes it's not enough. At times, you may be in a position where it's necessary to find complete strangers as potential friends.

- **Put Yourself in Unfamiliar Situations:** Putting yourself into situations where lots of new people are surrounding you at all times, and it's more than likely that at least one of them will stand out to you as a potential friend. This involves places like classes or work places. If you meet just a couple of nice people and meet up with them and their circle of acquaintances, odds are you will find new friends quite quickly.

- **Join New Communities:** Getting into brand new hobbies or interests, as well as joining new communities, is a great way to meet a lot of new friends. This will start friendships based on common interests so that you naturally have topics to discuss and things in common. You can find these by searching online for groups in your town.

To start with, getting to know strangers may take some extra effort out of your natural, daily routine. If a lot of your interests take place alone, you should find ways to get interested in events that involve more people. In addition to this, the simplest way to get to know lots of people is to be an excited person who engages in plenty of new activities and draws others to them naturally as a result.

The More People you Talk to, the Better Odds you Have:

As soon as you find yourself living a life where you have a lot of potential friends around you, you can figure out ways to start conversations and get acquainted with them in a deeper way. This won't lead to forming lasting bonds every time you interact with someone new, but if you put yourself out there often and find ways to talk to plenty of people you are drawn to, it's bound to happen.

You will even find that you mesh quite well with a lot of them. As soon as you have done this, you can confidently say that you have moved from common acquaintances, to friends. If meeting people and talking to them doesn't come easily to you, you may want to do some extra research on overcoming shyness and insecurity.

Invite New People to do Activities with you:

As soon as you have come across potentially interesting friend candidates who you click well with, you can approach the and see if they would like to do something with you outside of the current situation you are both in. This is a crucial step, and it's what separates acquaintances from actual friends. You can meet countless people and get along great with them, but if you never go beyond that and broach the subject of hanging out with them outside of work or school, you will never form deeper bonds with anyone. This will mean that potential friends stay someone you chat with only at work or school. You could be missing out on great opportunities by not approaching these candidates.

This may seem simple and obvious, but people who are more solitary by nature and perhaps a bit lonely can hit a wall at this point. There could be a person that they feel comfortable joking with at their workplace or even enjoy chatting with in between classes at school, but they are unsure of how to take the next step. In order to form friendships, you must learn to be the one who steps outside of this acquaintance level to attempt to make friends.

This may be more Difficult for Shy People:

If you are a shy person, this might be difficult for you. Sure, it's a little unsettling the first few times you do it, and you are risking that they say no, but you can get used to this quite easily, and you have to if you want to make friends. The plus side to this is it's a lot easier to ask a potential friend to meet up outside of school or work than it is to ask someone out for a romantic outing.

How Long it Takes to Invite them Out Differs Depending on Situations:

It depends on how you met the person, but you may end up inviting them to hang out outside of school or work quite fast or even end up waiting a month or more. For example, if someone you know brings a friend of theirs to an outing you go on, and you had an easy time talking to them all night, it may be totally natural to ask them to meet up again right off the bat.

In another situation, if you seem to hit it off quite well with someone at work, it may be hard to tell whether it's just a professional courtesy to get along or whether there is real potential for friendship outside of the work place. This may mean that you only talk every once in a while and don't know how to approach the subject of inviting them out with you.

Here are some Examples of How to Invite Potential Friends Out:

- **Make it Normal and Natural to get People's Contact Info:** If you desire to make new friends, the best thing you can do for yourself is getting into a habit of asking for new people's contact information early on in meeting. It's possible you could meet someone cool or intriguing, but you can't know for sure that you are going to meet them again, and opportunities are often lost this way.

Get comfortable with asking for people's e-mail addresses, phone numbers, or social media profiles. This ill mean that if another chance comes up to meet, you can easily reach out to them. In addition to this, if they also have your information, they can reach out to you to invite you to events.

- **Figure out How to Instigate Plan-Making with Others:** To get to know a potential friend, which requires hanging out with them, you have to know how to plan for it. At times, this is a simple and straight forward process. You request someone to do something with you, they say yes, you come up with a place and a time, and you're done.

However, other times can be a bit more complicated, particularly when there are a lot of people involved. You can have difficulty deciding on a place to meet or a time that works for everyone. You can keep in mind that there is always uncertainty attached to these events and that not everything is within your control. Trying is all you can do, at times. If you find that asking people to come hang out with you and trying to arrange plans sounds like a huge inconvenience, remember that others probably feel the same. Take turns organizing events with the people you know.

- **Try to Accept Invitations to go Out with Others:** Organizing plans with acquaintances is necessary and crucial to making friends, but make sure that when others approach you and invite you somewhere, you take them up on the offer. When we get into certain patterns of spending a lot of time alone or becoming workaholics, it can be tempting to turn down people's attempts to get us out of the house, especially if you are shy. You may find yourself tempted to rationalize reasons to stay home, even though you've really been wishing for new friends lately. Don't accept these excuses and force yourself to go.

In fact, this situation is even better than inviting others out because you know for a fact that person is interested in getting to know you more. There's no good reason to turn down a chance to meet new people and make friends. Who knows what this could lead to?

At times, you may find that you have to go through something inconvenient to develop your social circle and meet new friends. Maybe you will get invited to a show you're not very interested in, or someone might give you a call on an evening when you were about to go to sleep. It's to be expected that you will have to compromise at times, especially when groups of people are involved in the process of planning events. Regardless of that, these situations should never be avoided.

You should also remember that if you say no to many times to people's invitations, they may stop asking altogether. So, get out there next time you're invited somewhere.

- **Remember to Stay in Touch and Keep the Relationship Going:** You may meet up with someone once or even twice and consider them beyond an acquaintance level after that. For certain, specific people, this may be enough to be considered a friend. However, if you're hoping to build lasting, meaningful connections that go beyond the surface, it's not enough to only meet up every once in a while.

The more you see each other in new circumstances and the more you experience together, the better potential there is for growing closer and building a strong bond. This shouldn't be expected to happen with every acquaintance you have, but if you continue making it a point to meet new people and explore friendship possibilities with them, it should be only a matter of time before you make some close friendships that can grow into possibly lifelong bonds.

Start with the Foundation of Knowing a Couple People:

As soon as you have made a friend, or a few, you have a great starting point to build up from. If you are not really the social type naturally, this may be all you require to feel fulfilled. If you were feeling sad and lonely before, it will do wonders for you to have a couple of people to hang out with. Eventually, you will find yourself meeting with friends of your friends. If it turns out that you get along well with them, your social circle just got even bigger! It's also possible that you could become a part of the entire circle of friends, over time.

There's also the possibility that you can pursue meeting others in addition to this. Once you have friends, this will get easier since it opens the door to more events, opportunities, and new people to meet.

Go through the Steps Above Repeatedly to Meet even More People:

If you end up joining a new organization and meet a few nice people there, go to hang out with one of them and meet some of their friends, you have just taken a huge step in the social realm. However, if you pause right here and stagnate, that's all you will have. If you keep at it and come up with new ways to meet potential friends constantly, eventually you will find yourself with a lot of friends to hang out with.

It all depends on your personality type. Some people can have an unlimited amount of friends and feel very happy about that, while others would feel overwhelmed going past a certain number. It's all about what you feel most comfortable with. Don't forget that you can always search for more if you end up feeling the urge to do so.

Other Basic Principles to Keep in Mind:

Now that we have gone over the basic elements to meeting new people and making friends, we can get into other concepts that apply to the situation. These are principles that need to be kept in mind when attempting to understand social dynamics and build lasting bonds with other people.

- **Your Social Circle is your Responsibility:** A basic principle to making a group of friends is taking the first initiative. Some people make the huge mistake of waiting around for others to take the initiative to befriend them, invite them to things, and pursue a connection with them beyond work or school. Sure, that may happen sometimes, which is great, but you should never expect that or depend on it.

If you have made the decision that you want a social circle, come to terms with the fact that you need to make an effort to get it. If you are feeling active and desire to do something on Friday, don't just wait around for a call. You can put things together and be the one who invites others out. You can even call them up and see if they already have plans that you can tag along for.

Don't succumb to fears of coming across as needy or desperate. Remember that this is your commitment and you are willing to do whatever it takes to get out there and meet people. Remember that others may feel the same hesitation or apprehension that you feel when wanting to invite them out. What you put in is what you get back.

- **Don't get Offended if People don't seem Responsive:** Sometimes, others are preoccupied, busy, or thoughtless about attempting to hang out with you. This could lead to them never asking you to meet up and mean that you need to take the first step. Also, they may never think to invite you out if you don't take the initiative and get to know them better, first.

  On a similar note, some individuals are really laid back and lax about getting back to you over text or e-mail. This doesn't mean that they are trying to ignore you or reject your attempts to get to know them. It can be a simple personality quality.

- **Don't get Hung up on Thinking it's Hard to Make Friends:** If you are not used to making attempts to meet friends, you might think of the whole experience as complicated and inconvenient. After all, a lot of times, all you have to do is meet someone you get along with and make an effort to see them multiple times. You also shouldn't think that you need to get to know them for a long time before thinking of them as a friend.

A quality you will notice in people who are very social is that they will use that word quite loosely with people. This doesn't mean that those connections are always deep or very personal bonds, but you can still enjoy their presence and gradually grow closer with time.

- **Remember that you Cannot be too Picky at First:** If you need friends and have been feeling very lonely, your very first priority should be starting from where you are. This means hanging out with anyone who gets along with you and appears to be interested in you as a person. This doesn't mean that the first few friends you make will be ideal in every way or end up as best friends, but there are a lot of benefits to just getting out there instead of staying at home alone.

  You can also remember that you will find it easier to meet new people when you already have a couple of friends. Plus, if you are just starting out with creating your first social circle, it can be hard to tell what you value in friends. The only way to find out is to meet as many as possible. A basic rule you can apply here is that if you seem to get along decently with a person, making the effort to get to know them more can let you know if they are a potential friend.

If you are more on the picky side with social relations, you can find plenty of reasons to hold yourself back from making friends. But once you force yourself to hang out with them anyway, you have already gotten past this block and might find that you enjoy their presence more than you expected. People can often surprise you in this way and this can lead to lifelong friendships.

- **Try not to be too Negative about the Process:** Plenty of research has shown that people who are solitary or lonely by nature have a tendency to have negative attitudes about other people, more so than people with a lot friends. People who are not as outgoing have the luxury of being more selective with who they want to spend time around.

If you find yourself wanting to look down on people you meet, you should make the effort to look past these urges.

- **Take Note of your Imagine of Yourself:** A negative self-image can also contribute to being judgmental about other people. Work on making sure that your image of yourself is realistic and healthy, and you will go a long way toward making good friends. If you don't have the highest opinion of yourself, you may find it difficult to be around people that are a lot like you since it can show you what you don't like about yourself.

Try to take note of reasons why you might want to avoid new potential friends. It could turn out that you are giving up great opportunities to get to know nice people just because of your own insecurities.

- **Remember to Stay Persistent in the Process:** You may find that at times you join a hobby group or get introduced to a group of people with high hopes, and nothing seems to come of it. This may tempt you to become disheartened by the whole process and want to give up. It may lead you to think that you just don't get along with others or that they are rejecting you.

Do yourself, and others, a favor by giving the people more than one try. It's normal that the first time or two, you don't connect very well with people, but it can happen eventually if you make more efforts to hang out. If you find that a person declines your invite because they are busy that evening, don't allow this to make you give up on the whole process. Try it again later. You should never jump to assumptions about their attitudes toward you based on something like this.

With this process, it pays to only make positive assumptions. Even taking the initiative to invite someone out shows them that you like them and want to get to know them better. Just because they can't hang out that first time, but the invitation will put you into their mind for future events.

- **Stay Realistic about Expectations:** Remember that when you are just getting to know new people, you should stay realistic about how important you are to them. After all, they don't know you that well yet, and it's going to take some time to get closer with them. Remember that they probably already have friends and could be busier than you or occupied with other things. Don't expect that they will want to jump into hanging out every day with you right after you meet them for the first time. It could take a while to get closer to them.

At times, it won't end up being fruitful to try to get to know someone. It may appear promising at first, but then things could fizzle out after you meet up with them another couple of times. Either that, or they could be available the first time or two and then end up falling off the map soon after. This could be because they are busy with work, have a lot of friends already, or plenty of other reasons. You shouldn't take this personally and let it get you down. This is a common situation that everyone experiences.

If People Seem Uninterested in Getting to Know you More:

The idea of being the first to take initiative and not giving up right away can be all some people need to meet the perfect friends. Sometimes, even after taking initiative and persisting with people, you find that people still don't respond. There are a few things to keep in mind when this happens:

- **Stay as Patient as you can:** In an ideal world, you would find a great circle of friends very fast, even after moving somewhere completely new. You would meet your best buddy the first day after arriving to the new city or starting a new job. Unfortunately, life rarely works out this way. You will usually find that friendships take longer than that to form, but you should always stay with the process instead of giving up.

You may find that it takes a long time before you meet the right people who will be your close, lasting friends. Even after this, you may find that some months need to pass before you get to know them a lot better or see them often.

Even after that, it could take years to develop into very close friends who you will have for life. Remember that it usually takes some time to shift from not having plans, to making consistent plans with one person all the time, to having them in your life permanently or constantly.

Chapter 5: Strengthening Existing Relationships

Friends are valuable to us in life, and we all need them. In a lot of situations, they are what saves us during the hard times and give us the strength to persevere. Whether you are going through a divorce, the loss of a loved one, or another huge shift in life, friends will come to your rescue and revive your hope in life. They will be there to give you advice, new perspectives, and more. They will provide you with courage and strength when you have none.

Part of, not only making friends, but strengthening existing bonds with friends, is knowing how to analyze people and carry yourself. A friendship is not something that is simply created and then lasts forever without effort. A friendship must be constantly rebuilt and worked on, which is what makes it so valuable to us. So, the question is, when undertaking the quest of understanding ourselves and others better, and attempting to strengthen our existing friendships, how can we deepen these bonds?

Here are some Surefire Ways to Strengthen the Important Bonds in your Life:

- **Make Sure you Stay Aware of your Friendships:** At times, we become so busy and preoccupied with family and life that we almost forget that our friendships exist. This means that we need to stay conscious of these people and remember that they won't exist forever. Maybe they are just a classmate or neighbor at one point, but that doesn't mean they won't become closer to us later. Remember that whoever you spend the most time with is who you are working on building real friendships with.

- **Never Take them for Granted:** Remember that being friends with someone is a choice you constantly make, not something you are obligated to do. This is what makes it so valuable and meaningful. If you do not stay aware of this fact and value the people who are close to you, they won't stay close for long, unfortunately.

In our busy modern society, everyone is moving constantly. If we don't make it a point to pay attention to our close friends, they will get further and further away from us until we are left wondering what ever happened to the people we held so dear at one point.

- **Look for Ways to Help your Friends in Times of Need:** Having friends is great because we can rely on them to be there, but this means we need to return the favor and always look for ways to help them out of hard times. The best time to be the best friend you can be is when your friend is going through a hard time.

This doesn't mean you need to take it upon yourself to solve all of their issues, because this can weigh on you in a negative way, but you can be a listening ear and a shoulder to cry on, if they need it. You can be there to help them with errands or meals, if they need it, as well.

At times, people who are going through hard or trying times are afraid to impose upon you, so they don't reach out. This is the perfect opportunity to be the first to extend the warm hand of friendship and find out how you can help them, without waiting for them to ask you for help.

- **Look for Ways to Improve your Friend's Lives:** You shouldn't only extend a warm hand of friendship to your close loved ones when they are going through something difficult. Search for ways to make their lives happier and more meaningful. Maybe they are busy with work but need to get something else done. This is the perfect chance to step in and do them a favor.

Maybe they need a babysitter but haven't had a chance to call one. This is the perfect chance to do them a favor, without being asked. Always be looking for ways to help them out and make them even happier to be friends with you.

- **Never Forget Quality Time with your Friends:** Sure, this may seem obvious, but it's important to keep in mind. Family demands or work issues can take up a lot of our time. Daily schedules may seem like endless demanding to-do lists, but we must always make time to meet with our friends. We should set aside at least one day a week to spend time with them to keep the friendship growing and flourishing. Otherwise, we may lose them.

- **Make Sure to Stay in Touch all the Time:** Along with setting aside quality time to spend with your friends, you should make it a point to talk to them and catch up with them apart from this, as well. Not communicating with your friends enough will play a negative role on the relationship and must be kept in mind. We have the advantage in modern day of having devices which make it easy and simple to reach out to someone with a quick email or text. Stay in touch with your friends, even if it's a small message or quick phone call. This can make all the difference when it comes to your relationship.

- **Always be Supportive of their Aspirations:** You may find that your friends get lost sometimes, seem confused, or need advice. You must set aside time in your day to offer them the help they need. This is what friends are for. A lot of people in our lives are quick to laugh off someone's idea or passion, and friends should never be the ones who do this.

Friends should be there to listen to our ideas and give us encouragement when we need it. We should also be able to share our dreams with them and receive support back. If you want to make your friendships stronger and more lasting, you need to give them constructive, helpful advice that will be of value to their specific life path. There may be times that you find your friend's idea silly, but even then, you should help them make a list of pros and cons and find the best way to navigate their dream.

- **Remember how Important Friendship is:** The reason why we keep certain people around us month after month or year after year is because they matter to us in a significant way. Not having time is a terrible excuse to abandon your friendships. When something truly matters to you, you make the time, no matter what.

At times, we get overwhelmed and busy, but if your close relationships mean a lot to you, take the time to make them a top priority in your life. As soon as you do this, you will give yourself the permission to place friendship in front of other obligations that are, in reality, less important to you on a fundamental level. While issues or busy work schedules come and go, friendships can last forever.

At the end of life, it is not the hours we didn't work that we will look back upon with regret, but the time we didn't spend with the ones we love the most. Always keep in mind how important these bonds are.

- **Be Forgiving about their Faults:** It's natural that friends will get on your nerves at times with their habits or behavior. But, if they are a great friend, you should look past this for the sake of preserving the relationship. Everyone has their good and bad qualities, and true friendship embraces and accepts them all.

Sure, it may be hard, but to preserve the friendship, it's worth it to look past these qualities that annoy you.

- **Keep Expectations in Check:** You may find that when you observe your annoyance at a close friend, your anger is due to them defying an expectation you had of them that may have been unrealistic. We want our friends to call us every birthday, thank us for everything we do for them, and remember every important event in our lives, but fulfilling all of this is not always possible.

This kind of attitude can ruin a great friendship. Don't expect your friends to be perfect all the time. It's hard to find valuable friends, so once you do, keep your expectations in check and treat them fairly. It's worth it to save something that is so beneficial and worthwhile. If you treat them this way, they will return the favor.

Chapter 6: The dark side of human psychology – detecting liars, cheaters, and others alike

If only detecting liars was as easy as seeing if Pinocchio grow his nose, liars wouldn't exist in today's world. Sadly this is not the case and they are found much often than you would think. Detecting hidden negative aspects of a person's character can be tough, but using human psychology and picking up certain verbal and non-verbal cues can influence your relationship with that person of interest.

Verbal and Nonverbal Cues

There are many different ways someone can detect a liar or a cheater. In fact, many of the cues that a person will give off if they are cheating on their partner or lying to someone are actually nonverbal. This is mostly because the majority of the way people communicate are through facial expression, body language, eye contact (or lack thereof) and tone of voice. Research shows that 97% of our commination is nonverbal, while only 7% is verbal. Remember the old saying "It's not so much what you say, but how you say it"? Well, that stands true in many different cases. You don't have to be a detective or private investigator to spot if someone is being untruthful or deceitful, you just need to learn how to pick up on a few things.

It is easiest to do this when you know the person intimately, yet it can also be the hardest simply because of the emotions that are tied into it. You can't be betrayed by an enemy. Yet, it is usually best to know the truth. One of the easiest ways to know if someone is cheating on you is by their behavior. There are times when, on the surface, the person you suspect is lying and/or cheating on you will act as if they are more in love with you. Many times, because people do not know the signs to look for, people get away with cheating and lying, at least for a while, because their spouse or significant other does not suspect there is a problem. On the contrary, the one who is being lied to might think that their relationship has never been better. The one who is being deceitful may perform outward acts of affection, such as buying presents or taking their partner places, as a way to deal with their immense feelings guilt. They do this in an attempt to justify their actions to themselves. They will usually then have thoughts like "I'm not that bad, look at all this awesome stuff I've been buying her lately! She's lucky to have someone like me around, no one else would do all this stuff for her."

This behavior will go on usually only until the other person feels there may be something going on and begins to ask questions. At this point, the one who is lying or cheating would become avoidant or hostile. In some cases, the person who is cheating and lying will go through both phases, first becoming avoidant in hopes that they can steer clear of conflict. If the questioning persists, they may then become hostile in an attempt to place the blame on the innocent partner, so that they do not need to accept the blame themselves.

During the avoidance phase, the liar or cheater will usually not be able to look you in the eye when you ask them a direct question related to their activity. There may be long pauses before an answer is given and answers are either very vague, or they may get nervous and give out too much information than is necessary for that particular question. Intimacy and physical touch usually suffers and may become nonexistent. They may have trouble sleeping and eating, and may become very irritable when you try to talk to them.

Another way to tell if someone is lying is if they are looking at you, and then in response to your question or statement, they look down and to the left. Later on, during the hostile phase, the person's tone of voice will most likely be harsh and accusing. People naturally become defensive if they are doing something wrong and someone, in turn, accuses them of that wrong action.

Conclusion

Thank you again for downloading this book!

I hope this book was able to help you to feel more confident in reading people, interacting with them, and expressing yourself to strangers and friends alike. People struggle with this aspect of life only because they don't have access to the right information. Now that you have read this guide, you're well on your way to becoming a master communicator with fewer and fewer misunderstandings and mistakes in interactions.

The next step is to test out the information you read in this book for yourself and see how well it works for you. If you follow the facts given in this guide, you should see an improvement in your ability to read others and communicate with them within a short period of time. You can then pass along this knowledge to others.

Don't forget that the way people seem to express themselves is not always telling of how they truly feel, and that culture plays a huge role in body language and what it means.

Finally, if you enjoyed this book, then I'd like to ask you for a favor, would you be kind enough to leave a review for this book on Amazon? It'd be greatly appreciated!

Thank you and good luck!

Discover my other books in the "Psyched Out! Conquer Your Mind and Regain Your Life" Series

Book 1: Anxiety: Overcome Stress, Panic Attacks, and Fear. *Find Relief to Free Yourself and Most Importantly Unleash Your Inner Peace*

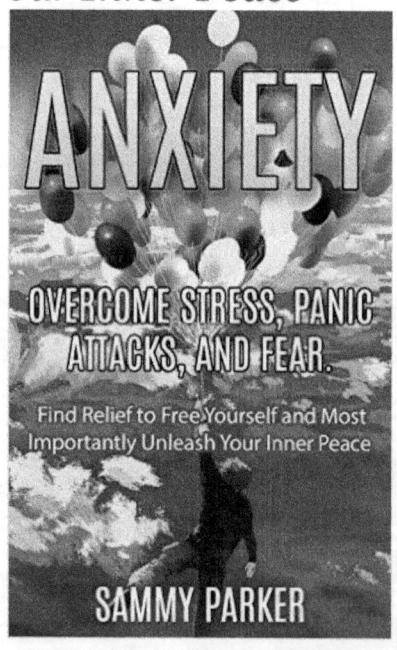

"The author also emphasized that it is really possible to win over anxiety. If you're anxiety is accompanied by stress, panic attacks and all kinds of fears, then you have have to heed the lessons from this book and gradually your anxiety will disappear." – Henry T.

Book 2: "Anxiety: Free Yourself from Shyness, Constant Worry, and Trepidation. Understand The Root of Your Emotion, What's Causing Them, And Why. Take Charge of Your Life, Conquer Your Fear, And Find Relief From Acute and Chronic Stressors

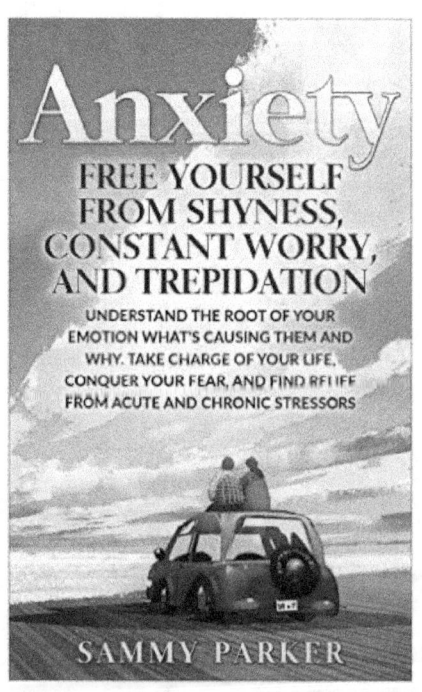

"Through this book you learn, roots of your emotions , common types of Anxiety, misconception about anxiety, implementing steps to defeat anxiety, conquering fear, and so on. The contents in this book is highly beneficial to everyone." – Edwin T.

Book 3: (Bundle) Anxiety: The Essential Guide to Overcome Stress, Panic Attacks, and Fear and Free Yourself from Shyness, Constant Worry, and Trepidation. Crush Anxiety Today (Double Book Bundle)

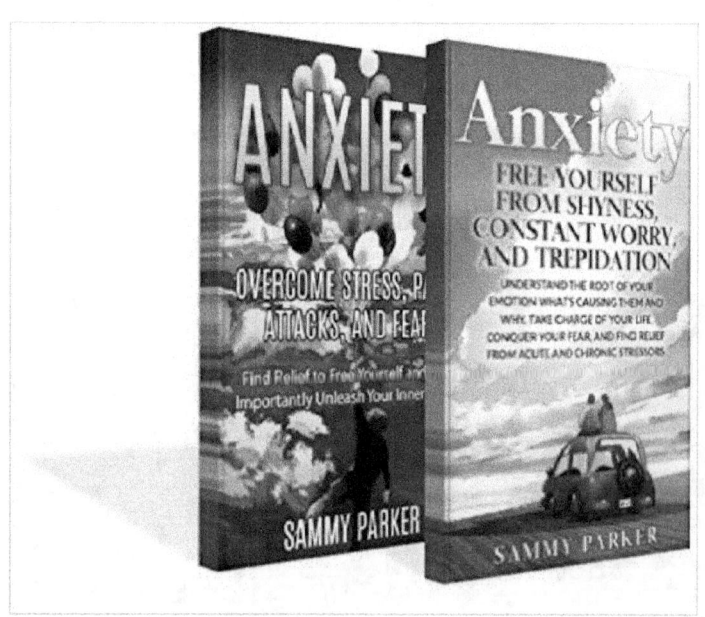

"This is the first time that I have read about types of anxieties, and the details are straight to the point. This book also gave me tips on how to overcome stress, which I will surely try. Great read, recommended for those who face stress everyday." – Krisanta I.

Book 4: "Depression: Naturally Free Yourself of Depression and Heal Anxiety, Panic Attacks, and Stress. A complete and direct guide to cure and overcome sadness, misery, sorrow and other factors that contribute to depression"

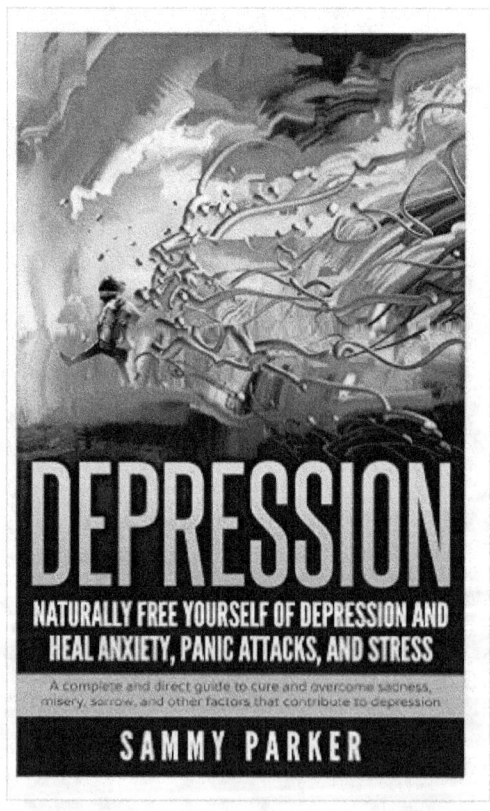

"This book explains how depression could affect our life, how it starts and some plans and guidelines to take action to cure it." – Spencer R.

Book 5: "Anxiety & Depression: 3 Manuscripts"

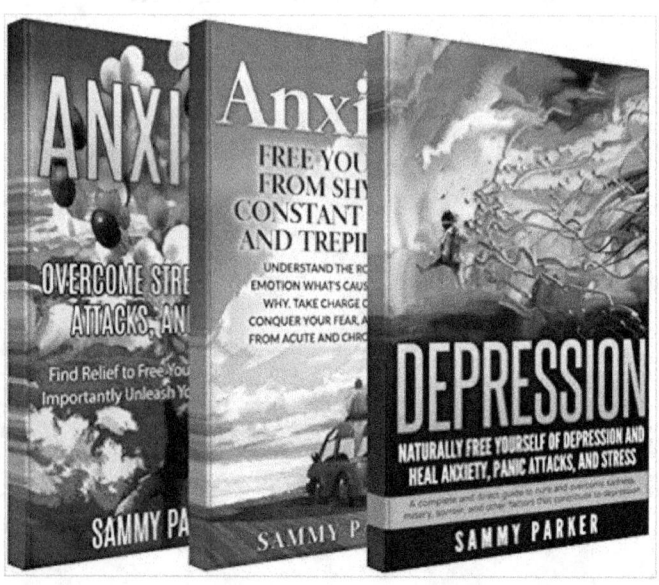

"This book explains what the signs and symptoms of depression and anxiety are. It also teaches you how to successfully cope with them and improve your mood. I highly recommend this book if you want to overcome your depression." – Ben

www.ingramcontent.com/pod-product-compliance
Lightning Source LLC
Chambersburg PA
CBHW070316190526
45169CB00005B/1641